PROTECTIO

The easy-to-follow guide to f
how to eliminate them fr
conveniently.

PROTECTION FOR LIFE

How to boost your body's defences
against free radicals and the ageing
effects of pollution and modern lifestyles

Dr Yuki Niwa and Maurice Hanssen

THORSONS PUBLISHING GROUP

First published 1989

British Library Cataloguing in Publication Data

Niwa, Yuki
Protection for life:
How to boost your body's defences
against free radicals and the ageing
effects of pollution and modern lifestyles.
1. Man. Health. Effects of diet
I. Title   II. Hanssen, Maurice
613.2

ISBN 0-7225-2197-9

Published by Thorsons Publishers Limited,
Wellingborough, Northamptonshire NN8 2RQ, England

Typeset by Harper Phototypesetters Limited, Northampton
Printed in Great Britain by Richard Clay Limited, Bungay, Suffolk

1   3   5   7   9   10   8   6   4   2

Contents

Contents

Introduction

Have you ever stopped to ask *why* we are suffering from more heart disease, cancers and degenerative diseases than ever before? Medical treatments seem essentially impotent against these illnesses, even though frightening amounts of money have been invested in the development of modern drugs. I've devoted my career to medical research, but instead of looking at modern synthetic chemicals, I've turned to nature for my inspiration. Here I have found the power to fight our modern diseases and the strength to protect us from our frighteningly polluted environment.

I believe that we can get the help we so desperately need from nature, without resorting to man-made chemicals that create even more pollution during their manufacture. Exciting scientific research carried out in the late 1960s and early 1970s started me thinking on these lines when it was discovered that oxygen can cause damage to the body as well as provide life. We have known for generations that oxygen gives life, but no one suspected that oxygen is also a factor in the development of degenerative diseases.

Even though my training and early career took me along the paths of traditional medicine, I discovered that my true vocation lay in the study of immunology, i.e. the development of disease and how the body fights off attacks from germs. I have thus devoted myself to the study of this area and have encouraged many young scientists and doctors to work with me to examine how to boost the human immune system. Together we have found a new way forward, a path that leads away from synthetic drugs and takes us towards certain plants and the enormous power locked within their cells.

I have discovered that a number of plants have quite exceptional properties in fighting off the damaging effects of oxygen. But unfortunately we cannot enjoy these benefits ourselves simply by adding the plants to our daily diet. What we must do is harvest the plants and then prepare and cook them in a very special manner. It took me years of study, of trial and error, elation and disappointment until I finally discovered the way to release the wonderful powers held so deeply within the plants. I found that the very best method is to use a special sequence of traditional Japanese food preparation and cooking procedures. The routine is far more complicated than the methods we use in preparing our normal meals, but it rejoices in the use of good honest ingredients (entirely free of synthetic additives), gentle but thorough heating, careful mixing, and controlled drying.

I'd like to share with you the exciting story of how I learned to harness the power of safe, natural plants and how you can benefit by boosting your body's ability to fight today's terrible diseases.

1
Oxygen: the common factor in disease?

Many people never give a thought to disease until they have the misfortune to detect a tell-tale symptom. The odd cough or cold is unlikely to worry anyone, but a sharp pain in the chest or the development of diabetes is far more serious. Major illnesses see us scurrying to our doctors for drugs and advice on how to cure the symptoms. But shouldn't we devote more time and effort to *preventing* the disease in the first place?

The upsurge of interest in health means that we are exposed to endless advice on avoiding stress, fatty foods, pollution, infections and so on, and there is no doubt that each of us can make some changes to our lifestyle to good effect. However, at the moment the human race is not winning the battle against chronic disease such as coronary heart disease, high blood pressure and strokes, rheumatoid arthritis, and cancer. I believe that we have been concentrating too much on trying to cure the symptoms rather than helping our bodies to fight battles against the agents that are bent on destroying our health.

I'd like to propose that the most destructive agent we have to fight is none other than that well-known element, oxygen. In fact, I'll go so far to say that I believe that 85 per cent of our chronic diseases are characterized by damage caused by derivatives of oxygen. 'Impossible!' I can hear you say. 'Extremely probable' is my immediate reply. I have spent many years working on behalf of the Japanese government, investigating the scientific evidence for oxygen derivatives as the destroyers of our health.

My research at the Niwa Institute of Immunology leaves me

in no doubt that, given the opportunity, oxygen derivatives wreak havoc in our bodies. Before I go on to tell you how this happens and what can be done to stop the destruction, let me reassure you that I still believe in oxygen as a giver of life. We all know that the air we breathe provides us with essential oxygen and that our bodies use this for those reactions which keep us alive and well. So how can it be so good and yet at the same time so bad?

The answer lies in the fact that the useful oxygen we breathe exists as two units bonded together chemically. The shorthand used to describe these coupled units is O_2. Bound together, hand in hand, the two identical units of oxygen are thought of as one entity and are scientifically described as a molecule. During the useful process of oxidation in the body, the chemical bonds between the two oxygen units are broken and the oxygen units are left frantically looking for a 'mate' to hang on to. It is this intrinsic energy that is harnessed and which releases the nutrients from our food, helps our blood to circulate, and generally keeps us alive.

The end-products of the oxidation process are carbon dioxide and water; each of these contains oxygen that is happily clinging on to a 'mate' of carbon or hydrogen. In other words, this is oxygen that is stable and not reactive. The body finds no difficulty in getting rid of carbon dioxide and water in exhaled breath and urine. But every so often a unit of oxygen is left without a mate; it cannot find another similar unit or one of carbon or hydrogen so it goes on the rampage in a frenzied attempt to seize a partner. It is at this moment, in a fraction of a second, that the damage occurs. The oxygen units that go on the rampage are called 'free radicals' or 'oxygen radicals', and may be denoted scientifically by the shorthand O_2^-, H_2O_2, $OH^{\cdot}$ and $^1O_2$.

It is when free radicals are generated in excessive quantities that tissue damage and disease ensues. Let me introduce you to a few free radical mediated diseases and disorders:

- arteriosclerosis

- cancer
- cerebro-vascular disease
- coronary heart disease
- diabetes (certain types)
- facial lines
- freckles and age spots
- ulcers in burns or wounds
- rheumatoid arthritis
- stroke
- sunburn
- ulcerative colitis

Unfortunately for modern society, there is mounting evidence that industrial pollution leads to the development of increasing number of oxygen radicals in our bodies. The sun has a similar effect, particularly as the protective ozone layer in the atmosphere is progressively damaged. Pharmaceutical drugs can produce free radicals as a side-effect to their purpose of treating the symptoms of a disease. What folly to cause a disease when trying to treat another!

2
The production of oxygen radicals in our bodies

To be fair, oxygen radicals do serve a very useful purpose as they are produced to destroy invading germs. The body has a good system for getting rid of excess quantities of free radicals, and in an ideal world oxygen radicals are produced as required and any excess is mopped up and made safe. But the human race has made certain that we do not live in an ideal world; we live in a world full of pollution, noxious chemicals, drugs, and solar/nuclear radiation. These hazards mean that we produce increasing numbers of free radicals and these add an extra burden to our bodies. To make matters worse, some people are losing the ability to mop up their excess quantities of free radicals. We know that older people are less able to get rid of unwanted free radicals, but research shows that many younger people lack the natural ability to fight the free radical invasion.

How and where are these free radicals formed in the body? There are five processes that generate free radicals:

1. Phagocytes
The word 'phagocyte' is derived from the Greek word *phagein*, which means 'to eat', and describes the white corpuscles in the blood that eat foreign invaders. Phagocytes are a vital part of the body's immune system, representing a first line of defence when harmful bacteria get into the bloodstream. Each phagocyte is a relatively large cell which literally engulfs the bacteria. Once inside, the bacteria are bombarded with free radicals which are produced by the white cell. In their highly excited state, the free oxygen radicals are quick to 'zap' the

invaders and destroy them without trace.

2. Radiation
None of us can escape radiation, although we are exposed to different types and doses. The radiation from the sun is one of our most insidious enemies. As we grow older, the skin on our faces and hands becomes loose and wrinkled, because the sun's radiation forces our skin to produce free radicals which then destroy the elasticity of the cells. Clothing effectively screens this type of ultraviolet radiation. A baby's bottom is often quoted as the ultimate in perfectly smooth skin, but that of an old person will often be similar, simply because it has never been exposed to the damaging effects of the sun.

More sinister are the types of radiation caused by nuclear reactions. The effects of the horrifying Chernobyl disaster will be with us for years as the fallout dust works its way through the food chain. But the human race isn't the only producer of nuclear radiation, there are rocks beneath the ground that emit radiation continuously. We cannot cover up to escape nuclear radiation, since unfortunately it penetrates deep into our bodies, causing the formation of free radicals with their associated damage and destruction.

3. Chemicals
This is where mankind needs a sharp rap on the knuckles. We have produced, and are still producing, far too many chemicals that result in the generation of free radicals within our bodies. To point a finger at a few, agricultural chemicals, Paraquat weedkiller, insecticides, anti-cancer drugs, and processed foods can be highlighted. Unless we move to organic farming and wholefoods we are all in danger. The formation of cancer is mediated by free radicals (see Chapter 5), so it is ironic that some of the drugs used to treat it actually cause the release of more potentially damaging free radicals.

4. Heart attack, surgery and strokes
Heart attacks, heart surgery, and strokes are characterized by

a period of time when the blood does not pass through the tissues in the normal manner. In the absence of oxygen enriched blood, the metabolic processes go awry and as soon as the blood is encouraged to flow once more there is a massive release of free radicals. The enzyme involved in this reaction is xanthine oxidase.

5. Metabolic processes
The enzyme xanthine oxidase is also responsible for the production of free radicals during the everyday metabolism of the superfluous components of cell nuclei. These components (purines) are present in the nuclei of all living cells, and excess and unwanted amounts are broken down and excreted in the urine.

The long-term toxicity of peroxides

In addition to the five processes described above, there is another system that generates free radicals of a longer-lasting and more sinister nature. These resilient free radicals latch on to the unsaturated fats that are integral components of cell membranes. They are known as fatty or lipid peroxides. The peroxides are not as destructive as reactive oxygen radicals in the short term, and are thus considered to be milder in their effect. However, in the long term they do irreparable damage to the integrity of the cell wall, encouraging ageing and the gradual breakdown of the protective cell membrane.

	Duration of action	Potency of action	Site of action
oxygen radicals	very short	potent	surface of target cells
lipid peroxides	long	mild	interior of target cells

Table 1 Comparison of the action of oxygen radicals and lipid peroxides

The discovery of illnesses caused by free radicals

Between 1970 and 1979 Yagi[3-8] was busy investigating the characteristics of lipid peroxides, and at the end of this period Boxer reported that a rare but severe form of anaemia was clearly related to an increase in oxygen radicals.[9] Boxer established that this increase was caused by a deficiency in the enzyme glutathione reductase.

Immediately after Boxer established the glutathione reductase link, I and my colleagues started to investigate the contribution of oxygen radicals to a whole range of common disorders. We were also keen to look for potential cures and spent a great deal of time investigating the effect of the enzyme superoxide dismutase on oxygen radical- and lipid peroxide-related diseases.[10-23] We also spent considerable time developing preparations of the enzyme superoxide dismutase that could be used clinically.[24-26]

I suppose it was a strange quirk of fate that at that time no one seemed interested in our discoveries. It was actually the work of biochemists studying heart disease and strokes in animals[27-29] that alerted the world to this incredibly important research. Now innumerable scientists throughout the world are busy studying oxygen radicals and lipid peroxides and their relationship to an enormous variety of diseases.

3
Illnesses caused by oxygen radicals

Medical and scientific research has established a number of links between the production of free radicals and the development of disease. I'd like to introduce to you the information we have so far.

The battle against germs

As and when germs such as bacteria and viruses enter the body, phagocytes cells muster to attack the invaders. The phagocytes are the body's white blood cells, and may be sub-divided into three types: neutrophils, monocytes, and macrophages. The white blood cells engulf the invading micro-organisms and then bombard and destroy them with free radicals. In some circumstances the production of free radicals by the phagocytes can become excessive and damage to the body itself may result. The free radicals are manufactured in the membrane of the phagocyte, and if they are not required inside the cell it is easy to jump out and seek a target for destruction outside the cell.

My own work on free radicals generated in this manner has revealed links with a number of different diseases. In each of the following cases the oxygen radicals are released by stimulated neutrophil cells:

Behcet's disease — severe inflammation of the blood vessels of the eye, ulceration of the mouth and genitalia and inflammation of other blood vessels.[11]

Kawasaki disease or Mucocutaneous Lymph Node Syndrome (MLNS) — a disease of small children causing fever, eye and

invading germs

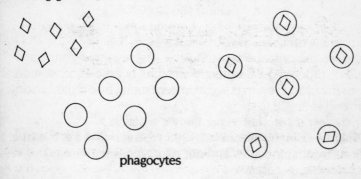

phagocytes

1. Phagocytes (white blood cells) attack invading germs.

2. Invaders are engulfed by the phagocytes.

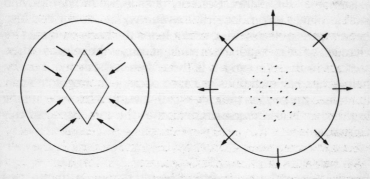

3. Oxygen radicals are generated to degrade or kill the invader.

4. Excessive oxygen radicals may be released and cause tissue damage.

Fig 1 The body's self-defence mechanism may generate too many oxygen radivals

mouth problems and swollen, red and peeling hands and feet.

Rheumatoid arthritis — where oxygen radicals are increased in the lubricating synovial fluid of the joints.[13]

Dermatitis herpetiformis — a burning and itching form of dermatitis with characteristic local lesions.[14]

Systemic lupus erythematosus (SLE) — a generalized connective tissue disorder, most frequently affecting middle-aged women, where the blood serum is active in generating free radicals from neutrophils.[15]

Severe cement dermatitis — an allergic reaction.[16]

Other work in my laboratories has revealed that it is the free radicals from monocytes and not neutrophils that are active in the following diseases:

Crohn's disease — inflammation of areas of the digestive tract.
Ulcerative colitis — ulceration of the colon.

The hazards of radiation

Radiation from the sun in small doses is essential to our existence on this planet. Not only does it give us warmth, and enable plants to produce the oxygen we need, but it is also beneficial as a disinfectant, and it helps the body manufacture vitamin D. The radiation from sunlight causes the release of free radicals in the skin, and it is these free radicals that can be helpful in small quantities or cause damage in excess. In small quantities the oxygen radicals kill off unwanted bacteria lurking in the skin, but in excessive quantities the same free radicals cause damage.

Skin cancer

In our clinics in Japan we often see old farmers with inflamed areas on the backs of their necks. These areas can develop into cancer if left untreated. The farmers have spent a lifetime outdoors, generally leaning forwards to tend crops or animals, with the sun beating down relentlessly on the backs of their necks. Generally, susceptibility to damage through sunlight increases with age as the body's natural ability to de-activate free radicals decreases.

Cataracts

Old people frequently suffer from cataracts which can ultimately cause blindness. It has recently been discovered that cataracts are caused by the attachment of oxygen radicals to the surface of the lens. Specifically it is the lipid peroxides that do the damage.[7,30,31] The greatest frequency of cataracts is found in Tibet where the land is high and the air is thin. Radiation from the sun has less atmosphere to pass through before reaching the inhabitants, so the danger is greater there than in less mountainous countries. Furthermore, the land is so high that there are few trees, so it is difficult for the people to obtain shade from the fierce midday sun.

Skin disease at birth

Some babies are born with a congenital inability to break down compounds called porphyrins that have been used in the respiratory process. A normal baby needs only limited amounts of porphyrins, but a newborn infant suffering from Porphyria cutanae congenita will have excessive quantities of porphyrins accumulating in the skin. These react to sunlight and produce a large quantity of free radicals, so many that the poor baby suffers from severe skin ulcers and associated skin damage.[32]

Freckles

People whose skin is prone to produce freckles know that their colour intensifies on exposure to the sun. The actual colour is caused by a pigment known as melanin. The biochemical process by which melanin is formed has only recently been clarified. Those interested may like to know that melanin is produced from the amino acid tyrosine, with DOPA (3, 4-dihdroxyphenylalanine), quinone, and indole as intermediaries. These reactions are stimulated or enhanced by the presence of oxygen radicals, which are produced in abundance in sunlight. It is interesting to note that vitamins C and E have frequently been used in the treatment of freckles. These vitamins have antioxidant properties and thus lessen the damaging effects of free radicals.

Sunburn dermatitis

It will come as no surprise to report that oxygen radicals are the main cause of both the initiation and worsening of this disease.

Radiation treatment

When someone suffering from cancer is given radiation treatment, the aim is to direct the energy of the radiation to kill the cancerous cells. This energy is mediated by free radicals, and these are aimed at the very heart of the cancer cells, at their nuclei. The nucleus of every living cell contains DNA (deoxyribonucleic acid) which enshrines coded instructions for the manufacture of new cells. The instructions on the DNA of cancer cells cause excessive cell division and thus the growth of cancerous material. During the process of radiation the nuclei of the cancer cells are bombarded with free radicals which destroy the codes so new cancer cells cannot be made. The great disadvantage of this method of cancer therapy is that free radicals are also generated in the nuclei of normal, healthy cells. It is this damage that causes the unwanted side effects of radiation therapy.

The unpleasant effects of chemicals

Free radicals are also generated in the treatment of cancer by drugs that are administered to stop the cancer cells dividing. Bleomycin[36,37] is an example of one such anti-cancer drug, others are adriamycin and daunomycin.[38-40] These drugs work by generating oxygen radicals in the nuclei of the cancer cells, radicals which then destroy the coded instructions in the cancer cells' DNA. Ideally the drugs should bypass the normal healthy cells, but regrettably a number of these are hit and the free radicals generated in the healthy nuclei cause damage to the material therein. This secondary damage is responsible for the extensive side-effects (iatrogenic effects) of anti-cancer drugs.

One of the main side effects of anti-cancer drugs is the destruction of some of the healthy cells that are especially rich in oxygen. Clearly the presence of oxygen enables the formation of oxygen radicals within cells. The drug bleomycin induces fibrosis of the lung as a side effect, so a proportion of the cells becomes fibrous and cannot function normally. The anthracycline drugs tend to affect the cells of the heart muscles as these too are particularly rich in oxygen.

It is desperately sad that anti-cancer radiation and chemotherapy can actually cause cancer in healthy cells as well as killing the original cancer cells. Just as oxygen radicals destroy the coded genetic material in the nuclei of cancer cells, so they can damage the genetic material of healthy cells. This damage to healthy chromosomes which carry genetic material can lead to abnormal cell division and cancer.

We must, therefore, start to take more care about our exposure to insecticides, drugs, detergents, and certain farm chemicals and processed foods as these are considered to produce free radicals in our bodies.[6,33-37] Exposure to or contact with these chemicals produces a surge of oxygen radicals in our bodies which lead to a variety of diseases in addition to ageing and cancer.

One chemical that has been the subject of detailed study is the weedkiller Paraquat.[33-35] It is possible to inhale minute quantities of this chemical on a regular basis until there is enough in the lungs to initiate a tragedy such as cancer or the birth of a deformed baby. If Paraquat is accidentally swallowed the situation is extremely serious as a massive number of free radicals are generated within the lung causing extensive fibrosis and consequent death. This happens because the chemical was developed so that it would destroy weeds by causing the release of free radicals within the nuclei of the plant cells.

Problems of blood circulation

When someone suffers from a heart attack or stroke or undergoes major heart surgery, there is a period when blood ceases to reach certain areas. If this deficit is left unchecked, serious and permanent damage will occur due to lack of oxygen (ischemia) in the tissues. However, with the correct care and encouragement of adequate blood flow, oxygen will return to the tissues and enable their return to normal functioning.

Surprisingly, if oxygen is withheld from the body's tissues for a *short* time there will not be a great deal of damage done. In fact it is the subsequent surge of blood (reperfusion) that wreaks havoc due to the release of large numbers of oxygen radicals. In cases of heart attack, stroke and heart surgery it is clear that the walls of the coronary arteries will have suffered for years from fatty deposits, and so it is doubly bad that the surge of free radicals when the blood flow starts once more, creates a considerable amount of further damage.

For readers interested in the biochemical mechanisms involved, the lack of oxygen during ischaemia causes the breakdown of the energy storage compound ATP (adenosine triphosphate) to its component purine nucleosides, and the conversion of the enzyme xanthine dehydrogenase in the blood vessels to xanthine oxidase.[27,29] During reperfusion, the xanthine oxidase acts on the purine nucleosides to produce xanthine and a large number of oxygen radicals.

A similar effect is observed in the action of stress on stomach (gastric) ulcers. One of the body's natural reactions to severe stress is to cause the muscular walls of arteries to contract, to make sure the blood is forced through to outlying muscles and tissues. If someone is suffering from narrowing of the arteries due to the accumulation of fatty deposits, any further narrowing due to muscular contraction can have desperate consequences.

People suffering from stomach ulcers tend to be of a type that are particularly susceptible to stress. A contraction of the arteries in the stomach wall can actually temporarily stop the blood flow. As discussed above, the lack of blood and oxygen for a short while does not do a great deal of damage, but the generation of free radicals when the blood starts to move once again can cause considerable damage in and around the ulcers. In this day and age of furred arteries, a small amount of stress can have significant consequences.

The contribution of metabolic processes

The enzyme xanthine oxidase is known to generate free radicals and it is a simple metabolic step to manufacture xanthine oxidase from its precursors in tissues such as the intestine and the pancreas. It seems feasible that certain triggers might cause the activation of the enzyme which may then be a causative factor in the development of disorders such as pancreatitis, diabetes, ulcerative colitis and Crohn's disease. As yet we do not know exactly what triggers the production of active xanthine oxidase, but such information would be particularly helpful in elucidating the development of a wide range of diseases.

Another important area of research centres upon the effect of oxygen radicals in releasing destructive material from lymphocyte white blood cells. This destructive material is termed 'clastogenic factor' and is linked with a number of auto-immune diseases.[48-54] Clastogenic factor is toxic to the cells of the human body and causes damage such as the breakage of chromosomes which carry vital coded genetic messages. For those interested, clastogenic factor has been identified as having a molecular weight of between one and ten thousand, and is inactivated at a temperature of 56°C (132.8°F), but is not inactivated by the enzyme protease.

It is known that clastogenic factor is released from the lymphocytes of patients suffering from diseases such as systemic lupus erythematosus (SLE), progressive systemic sclerosis (PSS), Crohn's disease and ulcerative colitis. The release of clastogenic factor is enhanced by the presence of oxygen radicals, so it may be concluded that these diseases are either induced, worsened, or both by the generation of oxygen radicals.

4
Long term damage from lipid peroxides

Although oxygen radicals are extremely potent for short periods, it is the lipid peroxides that do greater damage in the polyunsaturated fat-rich areas of the body such as cell membranes. Lipid peroxides are formed when short-lived oxygen radicals hit the fatty cell membranes.

Small quantities of lipid peroxides have essential roles in the maintenance of a healthy body. For example, the lipid peroxides derived from the arachidonic acids start the chain of reactions that activate white blood cells (neutrophils and lymphocytes) and blood platelets. This chain of reactions is known as the arachidonic cascade. The research findings from my own Institute indicate that the liver and kidneys have the highest lipid peroxide levels of all the organs and tissues of the body, suggesting that these are the prime sites of production (see Appendix, Table A1).

Problems start arising when the concentration of lipid peroxides exceeds a certain level. Yagi and colleagues[5] have proposed that the critical concentration is 5 nanomoles of lipid peroxides per millilitre of blood. He suggests that above this level the lipid peroxides migrate into tissues and organs to cause damage. This work, together with the findings of my own Institute, indicates that lipid peroxides are carried in the blood wrapped in a coat of low-density lipoprotein. This is the body's way of transporting a variety of other fats, cholesterol being one example. It seems likely that the lipid peroxides are released from their site of formation into the bloodstream where they are wrapped in their protective lipoprotein coat and delivered gift-wrapped to any part of the body. When they arrive at their destination they diffuse through the tissues and provoke secondary oxidative damage.

Damage to the arteries

Lipid peroxides play a major role in the development of strokes and coronary heart disease. To begin with the peroxides weaken the structure of the walls of the blood vessel, and then the little packages of cholesterol and fatty peroxides latch on to the damaged areas. These particles are known as LDLs, or low-density lipoproteins. Low-density because they are very fatty and have the tendency to float on water, and lipoprotein because they are a mixture of fat (lipid) and protein. The LDLs diffuse out of the bloodstream into the damaged areas of the lining of the blood vessel wall (the intima). Here they form foam cells which are considered to be the initial step of the thickening (atherosclerosis) and hardening (arteriosclerosis) of the arteries.[55,56]

If the blood vessels are in the brain, the strength of the walls can be reduced to such an extent that blood finally seeps through into the brain tissue itself. This causes a form of stroke known as cerebro-vascular bleeding. Alternatively, the LDLs clump together and stick to the wall of the blood vessel. This fatty deposit is known as plaque and if it builds up excessively causes the partial obstruction of the vessel. The next stage of the disease is for a small blood clot to form that cannot get through the narrowed gap, so the vessel becomes completely blocked. If the blood vessel is in the brain, this blockage causes a stroke (cerebrovascular thrombosis). If it is in the heart, a heart attack (myocardial infarct) occurs as blood cannot reach all the vital areas of the heart. See Fig 2.

It is well known that the weakening of blood vessels and the depositing of fatty plaque is a feature of our modern way of life. In fact, the build up of plaque (often called thickening of the arteries) has even been observed in young children. It is a disorder that develops progressively, affecting the vast majority of adults. Many a doctor offers the advice to 'reduce your intake

1. Blood flows freely in healthy vessel

No lipid peroxides in wall of blood vessel

2. Blood seeps through damaged walls into brain, causing a stroke

Lipid peroxides weaken the structure

3. Blood flow stops, causing a heart attack or stroke

Lipid peroxides deposited as plaque

A small blood clot can block the flow completely

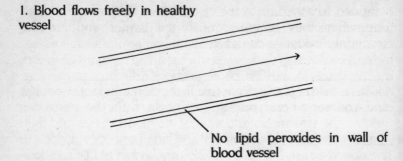
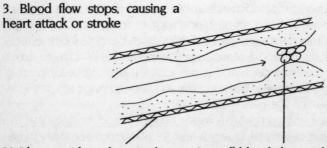

Fig 2 The role of lipid peroxides in strokes and heart attacks

of fats, especially saturated fats, cut down on cholesterol and increase your exercise.' In my opinion it is far more important to concentrate on trying to reduce the quantity of damaging free radical peroxides in the body so there can be no damage to the blood vessels in the first place. Without the damage there is nowhere for the LDLs to accumulate, so the arteries remain clear and free of obstructions.

Damage to the skin

The skin is constantly exposed to oxygen in the air and the ultraviolet radiation from the sun. In addition to the development of freckles and age spots and other skin disorders, oxidative damage in the skin can delay the healing of ulcerated burns and wounds and inflamed conditions or dermatitis. In my laboratory we have recently verified[21,22] that lipid peroxides are produced in large quantities in the damaged skin and slow down the healing process due to their toxic effect on cells. See Fig 3.

In areas affected by ulcers or inflammation with bleeding, some of the skin's cells from deeper layers are exposed to the air. Normally these would be covered by the protective hardened outer layer of dead skin (the epidermis). The outer membrane of the skin's cells includes polyunsaturated fats, minerals and water, all of which can react with oxygen in the air. Ultraviolet radiation from sunlight can make matters worse. Together the lipid peroxides from inside the body and the lipid peroxides formed due to exposure to air and sunlight cause further damage to the skin's cells. The production of these extra lipid peroxides makes it considerably more difficult for the ulcers and raw areas to heal.

Other diseases

Lipid peroxides have been shown to be positively associated with the lung diseases fibrosis, emphysema and bronchial damage. A number of studies show a link between diabetes and lipid peroxides. Diabetes has been induced experimentally through the administration of alloxan. It has been demon-

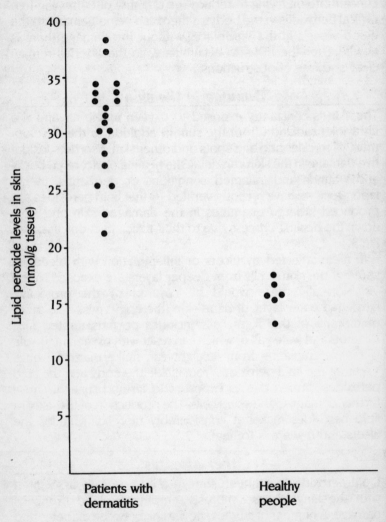

Fig 3 Patients with dermatitis have increased quantities of lipid peroxides

strated[41-43] that the diabetes develops because the alloxan stimulates the beta cells of the pancreas to release oxygen radicals in the nuclei of the cells. The nuclei are destroyed and with them the beta cells that normally produce insulin. Paraquat[33-35] and chemotherapies[36-40] have a similar action. Other studies[4,57] report that the lipid peroxides found in the blood of diabetic patients increase in concentration as the disease activity increases.

An increasing quantity of lipid peroxides in the blood has also been observed in certain cases of hepatitis where the illness has been artificially induced with the aid of carbon tetrachloride.[58] Additionally, lipid peroxides in the blood are increased in women suffering from the toxic condition known as eclampsia of pregnancy.[59]

5
Cell damage and cancer

There is no doubt in my mind that oxygen radicals and lipid peroxides are involved in the development of cancer. Everyone knows that cigarette smoking causes the accumulation of tar in the lungs, but it is not so well known that this tar leads to a steady increase in the release of free radicals. Similarly, the old Japanese farmers who develop skin cancers on the backs of their necks show a daily increase in the concentration of oxygen radicals. I believe it is the continued exposure to free radicals that creates the conditions conducive to the development of the cancers.

The cancer itself will not start to grow until the cells concerned suddenly mutate. This mutation involves the genetic material on the DNA (deoxyribonucleic acid) of the chromosomes within the nuclei of the cells. In a healthy cell the DNA contains the coded genetic information required for the growth, maintenance, repair and reproduction of the body. When a cancer develops the DNA mutates and starts issuing instructions to create lots of other cells in the immediate vicinity.

It is in the nucleus of a cell that Paraquat weedkiller, radiation and chemotherapy drugs such as bleomycin and anthracycline exert their effects. Each is a potent source of free radical generation, each releases reactive oxygen radicals within the DNA, leading to the impairment of the coded information on the chromosomes. The effect of Paraquat, radiation and drugs is dependent on the dose, the length of time administered and the health of the individual at the time. It is vitally important to calculate and administer the correct dose of radiation and chemotherapy drugs during the treatment of cancer in order to try to kill just the cancer cells and *not* the healthy cells as well. Extreme and intense doses of radiation or accidental poisoning with Paraquat can lead to death.

Lipid peroxides are involved in the development of cancer[47] as well as are oxygen radicals. Breast cancer in women has been linked with a high intake of cooking oils rich in polyunsaturates which implicates the involvement of lipid peroxides. Viruses have also been linked with subsequent cancer development, but in my opinion it is the oxygen radicals and lipid peroxides that do the damage.

The effect of age

After the age of forty the body's natural ability to get rid of excess free radicals starts to decrease. So the concentration of free radicals can start to build up, especially in the presence of an irritant such as cigarette smoke or pollution. With a reduced natural ability to get rid of the free radicals the older person has a greater struggle to ward off the development of cancer. This is why cancer afflicts many more older people than the younger ones.

Sadly, we are busily creating an environment around us that is conducive to the development of cancer. Our excessive use of farm chemicals, insecticides, detergents, drugs and processed foods is taking its toll. These are the materials that cause the production of an excess of free radicals in our bodies. Is it any wonder that younger people are beginning to suffer from cancers? Our natural defence systems were not designed to cope with the enormous amounts of pollution that we are now producing.

6
The body's defence systems

The enzyme system the body uses to counter the effects of excess oxygen radicals is known as superoxide dismutase. For convenience this is usually abbreviated to the rather unfortunate initials 'SOD'. Superoxide dismutase was discovered by McCord in the late 1960s,[1,2] following on from work on oxygen radicals carried out by Fridovich in the 1950s.

In most young people the activity of SOD increases whenever there is an increase in the quantity of oxygen radicals or lipid peroxides. This increase is known as the 'induction' of SOD. The same system exists in other organisms; plants can significantly enhance SOD activity[61,62] and certain bacteria have produced a twenty to twenty-five fold increase in SOD activity in response to oxidative stress from excessive oxygen and air pollutants.[60]

In every tissue and organ in the human body the level of SOD is adjusted according to the level of lipid peroxides present in the same site. This is a natural defence mechanism to protect cells from the potentially damaging effects of lipid peroxides. Table A1 in the Appendix shows that parts of the body with low levels of lipid peroxides have correspondingly low levels of SOD and sites with high concentrations of lipid peroxides have high quantities of SOD.

SOD is produced in the nuclei of cells in all plants, animals and humans. The enzyme has three main forms, each one binding (containing) different metals. The first contains copper and zinc, the second manganese and the third iron. It is the copper and zinc form of SOD that is the most important one protecting us from oxidative stress and this is the form I shall be describing hereafter. The production and regulation of SOD is controlled by the chromosomes, with the copper and zinc form controlled by human chromosome number 21.

Individuals differ markedly

I have mentioned that people over forty seem to be less able to cope with excessive quantities of free radicals than younger people. The response is related to the ability of the individual to induce SOD. I have recently reported my studies on the induction of SOD in old people and old mice,[22,23] showing that the older subjects were unable to produce enough SOD to counter the lipid peroxide damage in ulcers in burns. The younger subjects, whether man or mouse, showed a satisfactory response.

I have also mentioned that a number of younger people seem to have difficulty in coping with excessive quantities of free radicals, which is another example of inadequate SOD induction. In my work looking into the healing of ulcerated burns and raw patches in inflamed dermatitis I found that there was a considerable variation in the rate of healing.[23] When I looked at SOD induction I discovered that the people whose skin took longest to heal were those with the poorest induction of SOD. Those who developed SOD quickly in response to their increased levels of damaging lipid peroxides healed well. This work has subsequently been verified by Sugiura and his colleagues[63] who looked at the healing of skin ulcers. Sugiura also found high levels of lipid peroxides in the ulcers themselves, and showed that the subjects who were able to induce SOD in response produced satisfactory scar tissue. Those who showed no ability to induce SOD ended up with lumps of scar tissue (keloids) in their skin instead of a smooth finish. See Table 2 on page 34.

Smokers and lung cancer

My investigations into SOD induction and smokers add further weight to my theory that some individuals, regardless of their age, have a very limited or negligible ability to induce SOD. I

	Lipid peroxides (nmol/g tissue)	SOD (units/mg protein)
wounds producing satisfactory scars	24.4	20.5
wounds producing unsatisfactory scars (keloids)	26.3	13.8
healthy skin	11.0	12.6

Table 2 Comparison of lipid peroxide levels and SOD activity in damaged skin

have looked at 45 heavy smokers who have been puffing away on forty cigarettes a day for at least twenty years but had no obvious signs of illness. I looked to see how many oxygen radicals were produced by the smokers' neutrophil white blood cells, and how this compared to the SOD activity within their blood platelets.[10]

Most reassuringly, I discovered that by far and away the majority of smokers had the ability to generate sufficient SOD to counter their considerably elevated levels of damaging oxygen radicals. However, the results identified four individuals within the group who did not appear to be able to produce enough SOD to counter their elevated levels of oxygen radicals. Two of these developed lung cancer within 7 to 10 months, and, in retrospect, must have already been in the pre-cancer stage at the time of the study. It seems to me that this shows a pretty clear association and I propose that individuals who lack the ability to produce sufficient SOD when required are likely to be the ones who succumb to cancer.

In a second study[10] on smokers, I and my colleagues incarcerated 16 people for eighteen hours in a room with only poor ventilation, with nothing but playing cards for company. As in the previous study we looked at their levels of oxygen radicals and SOD. Everyone in the group showed a remarkable increase in their generation of damaging oxygen radicals during the eighteen hours. Of the 16, 14 showed a concomitant increase in protective SOD, indicating that they were able to counter the dangerous threat from the oxygen radicals. The remaining two showed no such increase in SOD activity, which worries me considerably as I believe it identifies these as prospective candidates for lung cancer.

The studies suggest that the ratio of the amount of free radicals to the amount of SOD is a good predictor of people who have a constitution open to the development of cancer. Those most likely to develop cancer are the ones who are unable to *induce* SOD to get rid of excessive amounts of damaging oxygen radicals. Smokers who have the ability to induce sufficient SOD to cope with the damaging load of oxygen radicals seem not to be affected with lung cancer.

SOD *activity versus induction*

Earlier in this book I mentioned that people over forty seem to be less able to cope with excesses of oxygen radicals and lipid peroxides. We must now pause to ask why.

If you look at the scientific literature, you will see that it has often been stated that older people have reduced levels of SOD activity, rendering them less able to cope with free radicals. However, Michelson[64] and my own laboratory[23,65] have recently discovered that the basal level of SOD activity is *similar in both old and young people*. That is to say, the level of SOD that exists in the old and young alike is directly comparable provided there is no need to get rid of *excess* free radicals that have been produced by oxygen stress. I confirmed this hypothesis by studying one hundred and sixty people.[65]

There seem to be very few people indeed who actually have a low level of basic SOD activity although as I have mentioned, there are a number who seem to have a limited ability to induce SOD on demand. So how can we identify people who are at risk from their inability to induce on demand this important scavenger of free radicals? It would be totally impracticable to ask everyone to puff away at cigarettes in a smoke filled room for 18 hours to check their response to their own generation of free radicals. So what can be done to identify those who need help?

Identifying those at risk

The widely accepted method of measuring SOD activity in humans involves taking small samples of skin or blood cells (neutrophils, lymphocytes, platelets and red cells) and carrying out tests. Such procedures have two drawbacks. Firstly, the assay of skin tissue and blood cells only measures the SOD present, when what we really need to know is the potential for the induction of SOD in conditions of oxidative toxicity. Secondly, the SOD activity assessed in platelets or red cells reflects the situation that existed a couple of weeks or months earlier than the test. This is because SOD activity measured in blood cells stems from the enzyme's activity in the bone marrow where the cells originated.

What we need now is a test that can measure the ability of this SOD to cope with the sudden increase in the concentration of free radicals that occurs under oxygen stress. We are actually working on a system to measure the SOD activity that will counter the excess oxygen radicals produced by the lymphocyte and neutrophil white blood cells. Once this is established we can start to identify which people are able to induce SOD in response to oxygen stress.

What will happen when we eventually produce a test that accurately identifies people who lack the ability to induce enough SOD? It seems likely that the best course of action will be to give them extra SOD to counter the damaging effects of their excess oxygen radicals. This extra SOD would help to combat our modern pollutants that act to increase the levels of oxygen radicals and lipid peroxides within our bodies. But giving SOD isn't as easy as one might hope — tablets of superoxide dismutase are not the answer as the enzyme gets broken down by the digestive juices and becomes ineffective. Injections have their problems, too, as you will see in the next chapter. I am quite convinced that we must follow the route that allows people to benefit from food components with SOD-like activity; this is why my work led me to develop Bio Harmony. Bio Harmony will be discussed more fully in Chapters 7 and 8.

Other agents that destroy free radicals

In addition to SOD, the body's enzymes catalase and peroxidase are potent oxygen radical scavengers. Oxygen radicals can also be destroyed by antioxidant nutrients in our foods. These low molecular weight antioxidants include flavonoids, polyphenols, catechins, carotenoids, vitamin E, riboflavin (vitamin B_2) and vitamin C.

Although oxygen radicals are fairly easily inactivated by these antioxidant nutrients, the fate of lipid peroxides is different. The lipid peroxides are produced at the site of the oxidative damage, and are then released into the bloodstream. Here they are wrapped in a low-density lipoprotein overcoat and sent to the liver for destruction. In the liver the enzyme glutathione peroxidase very slowly breaks down the lipid peroxides to alcohol and water. Even SOD is ineffective in breaking down the lipid peroxides. The importance of SOD is to prevent the formation of damaging lipid peroxides in the first place. The agents that will actually decrease the amounts of lipid peroxides in the tissues themselves are glutathione peroxidase or activated riboflavin (vitamin B_2).

Why some lipid peroxides cause damage while others do not

It is always a challenge in biochemistry to work out exactly what happens to products of metabolism in the body. At the moment we do not know exactly how lipid peroxides circulating in the blood get into tissues to wreak their havoc. At the moment the evidence that exists suggests that lipid peroxides behave in a manner similar to cholesterol. The work carried out on cholesterol by Goldstein and Brown[66-68] showed that the cholesterol is wrapped in low-density lipoprotein (LDL) before being delivered to peripheral tissues and to the walls of the coronary arteries. They further demonstrated that normal and intact LDLs can settle in the special receptor sites of the artery wall without causing any harm, prior to being taken into the cells for use as required. However, denatured or abnormal LDLs have odd shapes and therefore are unable to settle in the receptor sites. Instead, the white blood cell macrophages get hold of them and offer them to the inner lining (intima) of the artery wall, where they are taken in to form foam cells. As described previously, it is these foam cells that are the first step in the development of coronary artery disease. The metabolic pathway for the normal LDLs is called the 'LDL pathway' and the route for the damaged LDLs is known as the 'scavenger pathway'.

Yagi's work[55,56] has shown that lipid peroxides are delivered to the intima of the artery wall in a manner identical to cholesterol. It therefore seems likely that there are two types of LDL metabolic pathways for lipid peroxides, as there are for cholesterol. Those that cause no damage to the tissues will sit happily within the LDLs on their correct receptor sites of the artery wall. But the LDLs that are denatured or damaged will wander around until they can diffuse into the tissues without the mediation or proper control of an official receptor site. In this manner, lipid peroxides may enter the cells and exert their toxic effects.

Evidence from the human body

We have continually observed a close relationship between the concentrations of oxygen radicals and lipid peroxides in different areas of the body. It is especially difficult to measure the levels of short-lived oxygen radicals in sites other than the white blood cell neutrophils, monocytes and macrophages and the endothelial cells that line the inner cavities of the body. For this reason we tend to concentrate on measuring the quantities of the longer-lasting lipid peroxides and SOD activity in the range of organs, tissues and blood cells. Table A1 in the Appendix shows the quantity of lipid peroxides and SOD in healthy subjects.

In the skin, lipid peroxide levels are highest on the surface where they are in contact with the oxygen of the atmosphere. The activity of SOD is also highest in the outer layers of the skin, whereas in the deeper layers both lipid peroxides and SOD are less active. In general it seems that the SOD activity of the majority of human tissues and organs is equal to the maximum amounts of oxygen radicals and lipid peroxides that will be generated within that site. It appears that the more metaboli- cally active the site in question the greater the production of oxygen radicals, lipid peroxides and SOD. We have also ob- served this phenomenon within the phospholipid enzyme systems in cell membranes.[70,71]

There is some evidence that inside some of the internal organs lipid peroxides and oxygen radicals are produced excessively, that is, without the support of sufficient SOD. This indicates the possibility of the development of harmful oxidative effects.

Studies in my laboratory have confirmed that the various white blood cells generate differing amounts of oxygen radicals and SOD. Neutrophils are the most active on both counts, followed by the monocytes and finally the macrophages. In each case the quantity of SOD produced is sufficient to counter any excess oxygen radical activity. At the moment we have not shown equal activity within red blood cells,[69] but this is likely to be due to technical difficulties with the measurements.

7
The long search for an effective supplement

Having discovered that some people lack the ability to activate sufficient SOD to counter the dangerous oxidative effects of oxygen radicals and lipid peroxides, scientists worldwide set out to find a way to administer SOD in a form acceptable to the human body. This was not an easy task, and I believe it is important that you should know why certain preparations are worse than useless. Others are only applicable in carefully controlled medical conditions.

Injections

When SOD is injected it is extremely difficult to direct the activity to the sites in the body where there is an excess of oxygen radicals, lipid peroxides and oxidative damage. The SOD preparation has to attach itself to receptor sites on the outside of the cells at risk, and then penetrate the cell membrane in order to do useful work inside. The task is made more difficult by the fact that a mere six minutes after injection only half the active SOD will remain as it breaks down rapidly. After a further six minutes only a quarter of the original dose will be present, and after one hour only 0.1 per cent will remain. To make matters worse, most of the injected SOD tends to end up in the kidneys, ready for excretion in the urine.

One of the foremost authorities on protein investigation, Professor Michelson, has developed a preparation of SOD that can be injected with much greater success.[48,71-73] Professor Michelson's preparation is known as, 'liposomal encapsulated bovine copper, zinc SOD'. What the professor has done is purify

SOD from the red blood cells of cattle and suspend the enzyme in special minute fat droplets. These are dispersed in a watery fluid which can be injected into humans.

The advent of liposomal encapsulated SOD injections produced a longer life for the SOD within the body, a slower release of SOD, better total distribution within the body and the ability to reach organs other than the kidneys. It also greatly improved the fixation of SOD to the outside of cell membranes and enhanced its ability to travel through the membrane to the inside of the cell.

My own laboratories have confirmed the marked clinical efficacy of liposomal encapsulated SOD in oxygen radical and lipid peroxide related diseases.[24,48,70] We have also confirmed[24,74] that Michelson's liposomal SOD is effective in patients with severe rheumatoid arthritis, Crohn's disease, ulcerative colitis, intestinal Behcets's disease, mucocutaneous lymph node syndrome and the progressive sclerosis (hardening) or polymyositis (muscle inflammation and wastage) that develops with lung fibrosis. It is also effective in reducing the fibrosis following radiation therapy.[70]

A few people have questioned whether Michelson's liposomal SOD might lead to allergies because it is obtained from cows. I can confirm that we have injected more than one thousand people with the preparation and less than 2 per cent showed any adverse reaction. The adverse reactions were hardening of the skin at the injection site and the development of a fever during the first night. Blood tests from those who developed the fever revealed no evidence that they were generating antibodies against the preparation, nor was there any hypersensitivity. It seems probable that the acceptability of the preparation is due to its purity and the fact that bovine SOD is 85 per cent identical to human SOD. Bovine SOD contains no sugar chain and its protein loop is a beta structure. Proteins with an alpha helix structure tend to produce more allergies.

It is now possible to obtain SOD derived from humans by biotechnology, but we do not have any data to show that such preparations are actually effective. Professor Michelson suggests that a lack of efficacy could be due to the fact that human SOD would be more easily metabolised, and is not selectively bound to the sites where the excess oxygen radicals and lipid peroxides are creating damage.[75,76]

Will SOD supplements inactivate the body's own defence systems?

Intensive study by Dr Fridovich and his colleagues suggests that there is no system to inhibit the production of SOD in living organisms. This means that the body has no need to rid itself of any excess SOD — such a situation will cause no harm. In other words, if SOD is taken as a supplement the extra quantity will not upset the body's usual control mechanisms. It is fairly unusual that an enzyme system should lack such a biofeedback control mechanism; many others automatically stop natural production if there is an excess or if a supplementary dose is taken.

We looked at the activity in two other enzyme systems in order to assess the effects of SOD and antioxidants in cells. We investigated the activity of phospholipase A_2 and methyltransferase in the membranes of leucocyte white blood cells. Our studies revealed that SOD, catalase and low molecular weight antioxidants have no inhibitory effects on normal cell functions such as chemotaxis (the response to localized changes in concentration), phagocytosis (the engulfing of invaders) or the generation of oxygen radicals by white blood cells.

This work indicates that the presence of SOD and other antioxidants actually enhances the role of the phagocytic white blood cells in their fight against invading germs.[77] We were pleased to see that excesses of SOD and antioxidants did not reduce or neutralize the potency of the oxygen radicals produced to fight germs. In fact the presence of SOD and antioxidants actually *enhances* the phagocyte functions of white blood cell neutrophils against invading particles. This means extra SOD and antioxidants actually help in the fight against germs *and* get rid of excesses of potentially damaging free radicals.

SOD is useless in tablet form

Because the SOD enzyme has the high molecular weight of 33,000 it cannot be absorbed from the human digestive tract without first being denatured or degraded. It is simply too big to pass out of the gut into the bloodstream like other small nutrients. In fact a molecular weight of 5 to 6,000 is the limit for absorbtion from the gut without further breakdown.

An enzyme is an elaborate protein and is digested like any other protein in our diet. When it reaches the stomach it is broken down into small units by the action of the hydrochloric acid and the digestive juice pepsin. It is then absorbed in the form of peptides which are groups of the amino acid constituents of protein. In other words, when SOD is swallowed it is stripped of its unique biological function which is only present if the enzyme exists in its full sized, undamaged and undigested form.

So, why do we see tablets and powders of SOD for sale in Japan, the USA, England and other European countries? It is a nonsense to sell SOD in tablet form as the enzyme is only active if it can enter the bloodstream in an undamaged state. Injections of SOD are in order because the enzyme is introduced in its entirety, but injections are totally impractical for those who want to help themselves to health conveniently and effectively.

Harnessing plant power

What we had to find was a preparation with SOD activity (but not the large enzyme itself) that could be taken by mouth. People who are ill may be able to benefit from SOD injections, but those who currently show no signs of illness should have, in my opinion, the opportunity to be protected from the various diseases of oxygen toxicity. We need something we can take to ensure we have enough SOD to enable us to live healthily and beautifully, with reduced chances of suffering from premature ageing, cancer and degenerative diseases. I have personally been devoted to this cause for many years.

I had to look for low molecular weight compounds that would remove oxygen radicals and lipid peroxides from the body. We already know about the enzyme systems within the body such as SOD, catalase and peroxidase, but I was searching for anti-oxidant nutrients. I look at compounds such as flavonoids, polyphenols, catechins, carotenoids, vitamin C, riboflavin and vitamin E. These natural antioxidants can be found in plants and seeds, and serve the purpose of protecting the plants from the damaging effects of the sun. After all, many plants have no physical protection whatever from the sun's radiation, so have developed their own system for coping with the excesses of oxygen radicals released in their tissues.

Research in my laboratories showed that large quantities of antioxidants are present in sesame, wheatgerm, soya bean, Hatomugi (an oriental barley), Japanese green tea, Japanese Daikon radish and Japanese Yuzu orange. At the start of my research in this area, a good five years ago, I prepared various mixtures of extracts from these plants and fed them to volunteers. I awaited the results with eager anticipation, but to my disappointment, none of the mixtures was particularly effective and only one in five people responded at all. But I knew I was on the right track, and knew that I must continue to search for the key to release the active ingredients from the plants.

Then one day, quite unexpectedly, another experiment in my laboratory[25] gave me the clue I needed. That particular study involved separating out the plant components with a molecular weight of less than 30,000, and either heating these or treating them with digestive juices from the stomach. I discovered that after this treatment the plant components were *more* potent than they had been originally. The treated material proved to be better at removing excess oxygen radicals than the untreated original plants.

The explanation of this increased efficacy lies in the fact that heating and incubation with gastric juice releases low molecular weight compounds that were previously chemically bound as parts of polymers. These low molecular weight compounds include antioxidants such as polyphenols, flavonoids, tannin and carotenoids. In the plants, these antioxidants are trapped within the polymer structures and therefore cannot demonstrate their full potential. It is not until they are released from their immediate neighbours that they can start to exert their power.

So that was the answer. In order to extract *active* low molecular weight antioxidant components from plants it is necessary to liberate them from the confines of their restricting polymers. My next task was to find a method that was suitable for producing sufficient quantities of good quality material that could be made available to clinics and members of the public.

The ideal method

After a great many laborious, scientifically controlled experiments I perfected the ideal method. To begin with, the natural plants and seeds are stirred, slowly, gently and continually over a heat source. It is important that the heat should spread evenly throughout the mixture to prevent overheating and consequent damage to some parts, with insufficient treatment of others. I found that modern pans and ovens tended to produce a poor result with uneven heating, so I turned to the ancient Japanese cooking methods. The best results were obtained with a traditional Japanese wood-burning oven and an oriental clay vessel that spreads the heat evenly.

After heating, the mixture is brewed with Japanese 'Koji' which is a friendly fungus that releases large quantities of protease and amylase enzymes to help split the polymers into small useful antioxidant units. The mixture is then immersed in sesame oil which has been obtained from sesame seeds that have been subjected to the same method of heating and brewing. At the end of the procedure we have plant material rich in antioxidant activity and effective in countering oxygen radical and lipid peroxide related disorders. It is this material that I chose to call Bio Harmony.

The traditional Japanese oven emits infra-red heat which is particularly valuable in distributing the heat evenly. In combination with the clay cooking vessel, it directs the heat to the centre of the plant material, without denaturing or degrading the surface of the active components. Sesame, soya bean, wheatgerm and Hatomugi need this sort of treatment because they are rather dry and solid and are therefore not suited to a harsh form of heating that would tend to burn on the outside without their becoming warm in the centre. Additionally, a harsh form of heating would denature the important antioxidant com-

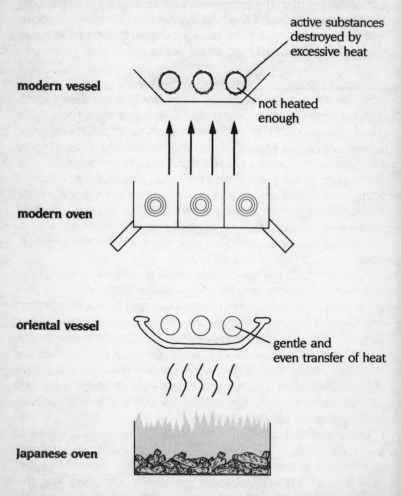

Fig 4 Comparison of modern and traditional oriental cooking methods

ponents, especially those situated near the surface. Our use of traditional methods ensures that the heating is carried out in a gentle fashion, at suitable temperatures and for optimal periods.

Steam treatment is used to prepare the green leaves of Japanese green tea, the immature leaves of Japanese Daikon radish and the Yuzu oranges. These ingredients are subjected to a blast of steam at 100°C for 15 seconds, which has the effect of destroying the unhelpful enzymes that can denature the natural vitamin C present, without destroying the vitamin itself. Leaves of the plant Aspalathus linearis, which is known as 'taste tea', are added at this stage to a final concentration of 20 per cent. Taste tea is especially rich in antioxidant flavonoids. The final step in the production of Bio Harmony is emulsifying the plant material in the specially prepared sesame oil.

The proof of the pudding[8]

In this chapter I'd like to present the scientific and clinical findings that confirm the enormous value of the specially prepared antioxidants that form Bio Harmony.

Effect on oxygen radicals

Under carefully controlled experimental conditions we looked at the efficacy of the untreated raw ingredients of Bio Harmony and compared these with the effects of Bio Harmony itself. In our study, oxygen radicals were generated by stimulated white blood cell neutrophils and by the xanthine-xanthine oxidase enzyme system. The results showed that both the untreated ingredients and Bio Harmony itself are effective in reducing the quantity of oxygen radicals. However, Bio Harmony is considerably more effective than its component ingredients in an untreated form. The statistical merit of Bio Harmony's efficacy in this instance is described as having a probability of less than one per cent. That is to say, its effect is so significant that such results could only happen by chance in one in every hundred trials.

We included a third material in the experiment as a control element for comparison. This control was a Chinese herb that is used as a medicine. Our results, summarized in Figure 5, indicate that the Chinese herb is marginally effective in reducing free radical activity, as fewer free radicals are released with increasing doses of the herb. However, this effect is tiny in comparison with the very marked effect of Bio Harmony in preventing the generation of oxygen radicals in neutrophils.

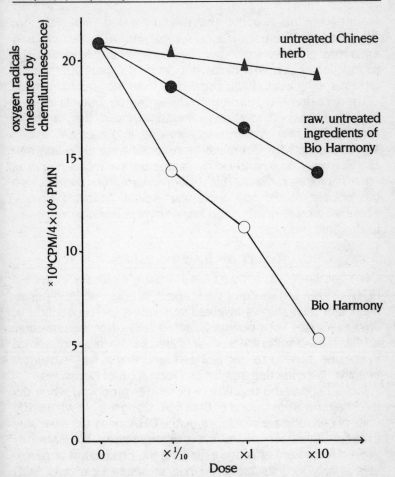

Notes for Practitioners: Chemiluminescence generated by 1×10^6 neutrophils (PMN) from normal individuals was assessed by scintillation counter in the absence of luminol in the dark (11-13). ×1 denotes therapeutic doses of each product (i.e. expected serum concentration after administration of doses, e.g. ×1 = 1.8mg/mg for Bio Harmony).

Fig 5 The effect of different preparations on the generation of oxygen radicals in neutrophils

In between the two are the raw, untreated ingredients of Bio Harmony. These show considerable antioxidant activity and are more effective than the Chinese herb in preventing the production of oxygen radicals, but clearly do not reach their full potential until heated and brewed to form Bio Harmony itself.

The fact that Bio Harmony reduces the quantity of oxygen radicals from both activated neutrophils and the xanthine-xanthine oxidase system indicates that it possesses oxygen scavenging activity. But much more exciting is the finding that Bio Harmony proved to be by far the most effective agent in controlling free radicals. This supports our earlier findings that the release of the low molecular weight antioxidant components through heating and brewing gives much more power to the final product.

Effect on lipid peroxides

Our experiments confirmed Bio Harmony's efficacy in getting rid of oxygen radicals. But what about its effect on lipid peroxides? Our next studies involved stimulating the production of lipid peroxides with polyunsaturated DHA (docosohexaenoic acid) in the laboratory. We administered Bio Harmony dissolved in sesame oil, and to our delight found that it was extremely effective in protecting against the formation of peroxides.

Table 3 shows the quantity of peroxides produced when different agents were added to the DHA. Using a scale where 100 units of peroxide are produced by the DHA alone we were able to check the efficacy of a range of different items. Bio Harmony proved to be very effective in limiting the production of peroxides as only 39 units appeared in its presence. Liposomal SOD was also very effective, but it should be borne in mind that this is the material that has to be injected so is not a practical alternative to Bio Harmony for the majority of people.

The raw untreated ingredients of Bio Harmony had very little effect in inhibiting lipid peroxidation. Similarly, SOD enzyme and water borne catalase were virtually ineffective. Other experiments showed that histidine and hypoxanthine were ineffective too. These last four agents are considered as active oxygen radical scavengers in their own right, but each was useless in coping with the fatty environment of the lipid peroxides. It is clear that the careful preparation of Bio Harmony is vital to its efficacy, and the addition of sesame oil essential to its fight against lipid peroxides.

It may surprise you to see that the antioxidant vitamin E has very little effect in preventing the production of lipid peroxides. Worse still, vitamin C actually makes possible lipid peroxidation so there is more damage with greater concentrations of vitamin C.

	Agent added	Index of lipid peroxides produced
	polyunsaturated DHA only	100
most	Bio Harmony in oil	39
effective	liposomal SOD	42
	vitamin E	83
	untreated ingredients of Bio Harmony in oil	85
	untreated ingredients of Bio Harmony in water	90
	SOD enzyme	94
	catalase enzyme	105
ineffective	vitamin C	136

Notes for Practitioners: Lipid peroxidation was performed by producing TBA reactivity[3] induced in the presence of docosahexaenoic acid (DHA) under ultraviolet light.[30] TBA reactivity was assessed using a spectrophotometer, measuring the absorbance at 535 nm.[3]

Table 3 Effect on the production of lipid peroxides

Added value

All my investigations indicate that the product Bio Harmony is far more efficacious than the simple sum of its components. I was keen to find out which particular active components, if any, were increased during the heating and brewing of the plant material. I decided to look at the following low molecular weight antioxidant compounds: riboflavin (vitamin B₂), vitamin E, carotene and tannin. For those readers who are interested, the scientific methods I used for this study were paper chromatographic and lumiflavin fluorescent analyses.

The results of the various studies showed that there were increases in several low molecular weight antioxidants during the heating of the plant components and their brewing with 'Koji'. The most marked increase was observed with riboflavin. At the other end of the scale was vitamin E which showed no significiant increase at all. These results (shown in Table 4) provided me with the clear evidence that the heating and brewing processes involved in the preparation of Bio Harmony do indeed increase the concentration of active antioxidants.

	riboflavin	vit E	carotene	tannin
raw ingredients	0.14 (mg)	0.087 (mg)	0.12 (mg)	0.6 (mg)
after heating	0.21	0.12	0.20	1.1
after brewing with 'Koji'	0.18	0.10	0.16	1.1
after both heating and brewing with 'Koji'	0.53	0.15	0.27	1.6

Notes for practitioners: These data apply to a single sachet (3g) of Bio Harmony. Vitamin E (alpha tocopherol), riboflavin (vitamin B₂) and tannin (catechin) were assessed with HPLC, and carotene with the visible absorption method.

Table 4   Comparison of the quantity of antioxidants present during the preparation of Bio Harmony

Freckles and inflammation

We have already discussed how free radicals are involved in the formation of freckles and age spots. You will recall that the effect of radiation from the sun on the skin causes the production of free radicals which, in turn, are involved in the generation of melanin. It is the brown coloured pigment melanin that concentrates in areas on the skin to give rise to the freckles and age spots. I can now confirm that Bio Harmony is clinically effective in reducing these skin pigmentations.[78,79] Melanin is formed after a series of enzyme-activated reactions, starting with the enzyme tyrosinase. Laboratory studies with Bio Harmony

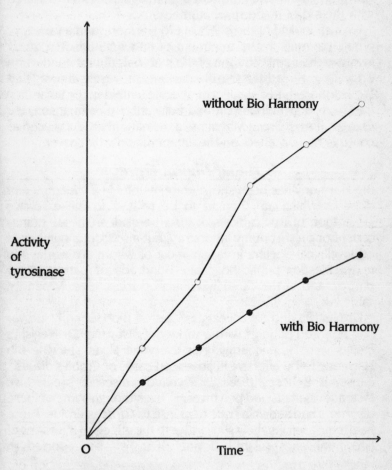

Notes for Practitioners: Tyrosinase activity was assessed by spectrophotometer at 475 nm, pH 6.8, 37°C, with L-Dopa as the substrate in a phosphate buffer.

Fig 6 Effect of Bio Harmony on tyrosinase activity

revealed that it effectively reduces tyrosinase activity, which in turn would reduce the production of melanin. Figure 6 shows how tyrosinase activity is reduced by a therapeutic dose of Bio Harmony. In this study the activity of the enzyme was measured with the aid of a spectrophotometer.

We also looked at the effect of Bio Harmony and a variety of other materials in the treatment of inflammation. The study involved the administration of the materials after the induction of swelling with adriamycin or adjuvant. The results showed that Bio Harmony had a significant effect in inhibiting the inflammation from both adriamycin and adjuvant. By comparison, the Chinese herbs, Green Magma and the natural products used as controls had no effect on the inflammation whatsoever.

Striking clinical efficacy

Bio Harmony has been shown to be helpful in a wide range of diseases which are thought to be related to the excessive generation of free radicals or lipid peroxides. These findings come not only from my laboratory, but also from a number of other clinical doctors in Japan, most of whom are working in universities or public hospitals. Hundreds of patients have participated in the carefully controlled trials. (See Appendix, Table A2.)

Dr Negishi and his colleagues[80] tested Bio Harmony in over one hundred patients with a variety of disorders. Dr Negishi's results were as encouraging as everyone else's, showing Bio Harmony to be effective in advanced cases of Crohn's disease, intestinal Behcet's disease, Raynaud's disease, progressive systemic sclerosis and polymyositis, even though some of these disorders had shown a poor response to corticosteroids. These heartening results show similarities to the effects of injections of liposomal encapsulated bovine SOD,[24,70,74] as reported in Chapter 7.

I'd like to tell you about some individual patients whose response to Bio Harmony brought them great relief and gave me considerable encouragement.

Four patients with Crohn's disease and ulcerative colitis with intestinal ulcers took Bio Harmony for two or three months. Previously they had had a number of surgical operations to remove parts of their raw and bleeding intestines, but had not been relieved of their troublesome symptoms. It was wonderful to see them improve with a course of Bio Harmony. I am delighted to say that before long they showed complete remission and required no further removal and resection of their intestines.

Three other patients had advanced progressive systemic sclerosis (hardening and thickening of the skin and organs) with widespread skin eruption, polymyositis (muscle inflammation and wastage) and difficulty in breathing due to lung fibrosis. They had proved resistant to all therapies including low dose steroids and the anti-tumour agent leukerin. One month after starting a course of Bio Harmony their difficulty in breathing had improved and after three months the chest x-rays showed a marked decrease in the fibrotic shadows on the lungs.

Patients suffering from rheumatoid arthritis also showed an improvement with Bio Harmony treatment which was especially helpful in relieving morning stiffness. One particular patient arrived at our hospital in a wheel chair as she was so immobile. She was suffering from swollen, painful and deformed fingers, hands and knees and was resistant to all previous attempted therapies. She had been treated, without success, with nonsteroid anti-inflammatory drugs and low dose steroids. We gave her a course of Bio Harmony and within six to seven weeks she began to be able to walk around with the aid of crutches. A few weeks later she was able to discard the crutches and walk unaided, albeit with a bit of a limp.

Figure 7 charts the progress of our plucky patient (who, incidentally, was only thirty four years old). Before receiving Bio Harmony she was on two drugs, Fenbufen and Piroxicam, and had marked symptoms of pain, swelling and morning stiffness. Her lipid peroxide levels had risen steadily over the preceding

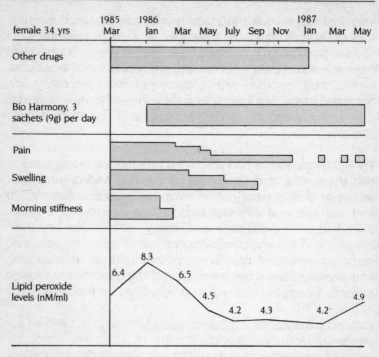

Fig 7 Effect of Bio Harmony on a patient with rheumatoid arthritis

ten months, from 6.4 to 8.3 nanomoles per millilitre. These lipid peroxide levels started to fall dramatically as soon as she started on her course of three sachets (9g) of Bio Harmony each day.

Within three months her symptoms had improved dramatically and continued to do so with Bio Harmony. As you will see from the diagram we continued to give her the other drugs for one year, to make sure the effects we were measuring were a direct result of Bio Harmony and nothing to do with withdrawal symptoms from her other drugs. After one year we stopped her old drugs and she took Bio Harmony alone. I am delighted to say that she continued to enjoy her new health, remaining virtually free of her previous painful symptoms.

Some of the patients with inflammation of the kidneys (nephritis) showed a marked improvement in kidney function, and some of those suffering from hepatitis showed an improvement which could be measured by a reduction in the activity of the enzyme system serum transaminase. Bio Harmony was also found to be beneficial to people suffering from shoulder stiffness, hangover, general malaise and other non-specific complaints.

Rather unexpectedly, we found that the common wart responded magnificently to treatment with Bio Harmony. Almost without exception a complete cure was effected from this tiresome affliction. This may be compared with the observation that chronic and severe viral eruptions such as herpes zoster and chicken pox tend to proliferate in areas of skin normally exposed to the sun.[81-83] It is known that oxygen radicals and lipid peroxides are generated in large amounts in sun-exposed areas, and it is logical to suggest that the structure of the tissues becomes damaged, thus reducing the ability of the skin to fight off an invading virus.

Improving blood circulation

Patients complaining of cold fingers and toes responded well to a course of Bio Harmony, perhaps because of its effect in reducing lipid peroxidation in the lining of the blood vessel walls.[55,56] Undefined chilliness of the fingers and toes can develop into the more serious Raynaud's disease. We were delighted to see that Bio Harmony is outstandingly effective in improving Reynaud's disease, especially as liposomal SOD injections had shown little effect.[24,70,74]

Bio Harmony appears to be remarkably effective in improving blood circulation. Its ability to clear the blood vessels allows the blood to flow more freely. As Bio Harmony also prevents the formation of new lipid peroxides it acts to keep the blood vessels clear in future. These dual effects ensure that the blood may circulate strongly and freely. Our trials indicate that Bio Harmony is frequently effective in reducing the quantity of lipid peroxides circulating within the blood itself.

Bio Harmony's ability to improve blood circulation explains its striking and wide-ranging effectiveness in improving a variety of disorders. For example, its action to lessen shoulder stiffness and the pain of lumbago may be assigned to its ability to improve blood circulation. Its value in treating a hangover can also be related to improved circulation, which hastens the removal of alcohol from the body.

Improved circulation is the likely explanation for the surprising finding that Bio Harmony helped women suffering from irregular periods. A number of women found that their periods returned to normal after a course of treatment. It seems likely that any damaged organ or tissue will benefit from improved blood circulation and this is probably how Bio Harmony helped the women. The potential of the material seems endless; so many disorders are caused by damaged tissues or organs, each of which could be aided by an increase in the blood flow reaching the area.

It should be borne in mind that lipid peroxides are not reduced by enzymes such as SOD (although this is effective in removing free radicals). Instead, the enzyme glutathione peroxidase has to go to work on the lipid peroxides to render them harmless. The activity of glutathione peroxidase is dependent upon the presence of riboflavin (vitamin B_2). This could be why Bio Harmony is so effective in countering the lipid peroxides; as riboflavin is markedly increased during the heating and brewing part of its preparation. The other important factor is the final emulsification of Bio Harmony in heated sesame oil, as this enables the preparation to get physically closer to the lipid peroxides instead of remaining in the water-soluble phase.

Encouraging progress

I am not going to claim that Bio Harmony is a universal cure-all, as clearly such a claim would be absurd. However, Bio Harmony has proved extremely valuable in illnesses with no effective treatment to date. These illnesses include Raynaud's disease and the lung fibrosis of advanced progressive systemic sclerosis and polymyositis. Trials have been conducted throughout the world with similar encouraging results.

In the treatment of liver disease, kidney disease and the cosmetic problem of freckles I wouldn't like to claim a success rate of more than 50 per cent for Bio Harmony in clearing all the symptoms. But, my goodness, what encouraging progress! Here we are talking of disorders that have shown amazing resistance to all previous attempted cures, and here we have a product that is helpful in up to half of these chronic cases. Table A2 in the Appendix summarizes the efficacy of Bio Harmony in treating a wide range of disorders.

What is so reassuring is the fact that Bio Harmony is made up of entirely natural ingredients, so it is safe to take and totally free of the frightening side-effects that accompany so many of today's modern drugs.

Anti-ageing effects

There is considerable evidence to indicate that lines and wrinkles are caused by an increase in the level of free radicals and lipid peroxides in the affected part of the skin. The radicals and peroxides are believed to affect the supportive network of collagen tissue, as well as lowering the skin's natural moisturizing ability. The substance hyaluronic acid, which is known to be an effective moisturizer, has recently been found to possess remarkable potency to scavenge free radicals[84] and render them harmless. Hyaluronic acid is actually a jelly-like substance that is extremely effective in holding water in the spaces between the cells. It also has a role in the human body in lubricating the joints between bones. In order to prevent ageing we need to keep our collagen in its youthful soft form (rather than the tough cross-linked form of later years) and maintain our supplies of moisturizing hyaluronic acid.

We know that free radicals and lipid peroxides proliferate in parts of the skin exposed to the sun such as the face and hands. With time, our supplies of collagen and hyaluronic acid become less effective as they battle against constant bombardment from and destruction by the sun. What is needed to prevent the development of lines and wrinkles are agents that will destroy the radicals and peroxides before they can do their damage. When we are young our supplies of SOD and glutathione peroxidase fight off the attacks successfully, but as we grow older our bodies need a little help. I believe that Bio Harmony can provide that help. I have talked at length of its efficacy in scavenging free radicals and destroying lipid peroxides, and of its acceptability to the body due to its being entirely natural. If you take Bio Harmony regularly you are giving your body a chance to keep up the work of its youth and to fight off damaging invaders effectively and constantly.

9
A promising outlook

There is mounting evidence that we have blundered on thought-lessly to create a world that is laden with industrial pollution. The air we breathe is full of noxious chemicals that are sufficiently reactive to cause the production of free radicals and lipid peroxides within our bodies. In addition, our wanton use of chlorofluoro-carbons (CFCs) in pressurized sprays and refrigerant coolants has caused the enormous hole in the ozone layer that is such a worry to us, our children and our grand-children. This hole allows more of the sun's radiation to reach the earth's surface, and increased radiation results in greater quantities of oxygen radicals and lipid peroxides in our bodies. We are going to need all the help we can get.

Can our foods alone protect us?

It is unwise to try to fight the effects of man-made chemicals with man-made drugs. The drugs themselves tend to have a lot of side-effects and there is a wealth of evidence to show that the human body does not take kindly to a wide range of administered drugs. There is no doubt that we do need help, and I am enormously encouraged with my scientific studies that show that help can come from *natural* sources.

Some people might query whether foods themselves could afford as much protection as a natural product such as Bio Harmony. For instance, many nationalities eat soya beans, sesame seeds and wheatgerm every day. Does this mean they enjoy extra resistance to the damaging effects of free radicals? After all, soya beans, sesame seeds and wheatgerm are among

the ingredients of Bio Harmony. The answer is that the foods
themselves cannot offer the same benefits. All foods are broken
down in the digestive tract into units that are small enough to
be absorbed into the blood stream for distribution and assimi-
lation. It seems that the body does not break down the foods
into the same sub-units as those found in Bio Harmony. In other
words, the products of food digestion do not reach their full
potential as antioxidants in the body.

All my work confirms that you *cannot obtain the full benefit of
antioxidants simply by eating foods in their natural state.* The heating,
brewing and lipophilization procedures employed during the
preparation of Bio Harmony are essential to allow the natural
antioxidants to attain their full protective and therapeutic
potential. And, incidentally, the current fashion of eating raw
food diets makes it more difficult for the body to obtain the full
value of a number of ingredients.

Are other supplements beneficial?

In theory it would be possible to make up an effective antioxidant cocktail from plant components such as flavonoids, polyphenols, catechins, carotenoids, riboflavin and vitamins C and
E. These are the low molecular weight active ingredients of Bio
Harmony. It would be a lengthy and expensive procedure to
isolate these compounds and then reassemble them, so why
not use a natural product in the first place?

It is possible to buy a whole range of synthetic nutrients, and
many people assume that these are as good as the original
natural varieties. However, the human body has a large number
of cells that accept certain compounds but reject others. It is
true to say that these cells show a far better affinity for natural
compounds than for synthetic ones. This is probably due to the
fact that the cells have evolved over the millennia and have long
accepted natural corns and seeds. Why should they now
change in the space of a couple of generations in order to
accept man-made nutrients?

I believe it is important to consume a range of nutrients at one
time. Taken in isolation, some nutrients could have the wrong

effect. For example, vitamin C is an antioxidant, but if consumed in huge quantities it can actually *increase* the production of dangerous oxygen radicals and lipid peroxides. It is well established that very high concentrations of vitamin C can lead to the production of large quantities of oxygen radicals through a reaction involving iron. During the process (known as a Fenton-type reaction) the iron is reduced from the ferric form to the ferrous form[91,92] and large amounts of the free radical OH˙ are released. Work in my own laboratory indicates that the presence of vitamin E and other antioxidants actually inhibit this unwanted reaction with iron. I feel this is a very clear example of the fact that the selection of one antioxidant at a time can be counter-productive. We need balance in all aspects of our life, including nutrients.

I find myself questioning why people buy chemically synthesized individual antioxidants such as vitamins C and E, riboflavin, flavonoids and selenium, apparently with the aim of improving their health. In our cultivated modern life there are few people in whom individual nutrients are selectively deficient. For example, not too long ago there was a remote mountain region in China, Keshan, where the diet was extremely low in selenium, which resulted in the production of excessive quantities of free radicals which in turn caused disease. But this was exceptional and was capable of control through nutritional supplementation. We do not tend to suffer from individual deficiency diseases today, so why select nutrients individually as though we do? I can see no point in continuing along the single-nutrient supplement path. After all, no one can say that it has cured our ailments or made us super healthy. There are, of course, manufacturers who produce balanced supplements from naturally-sourced raw materials which can have a useful role and are far superior to the single synthetic nutrients.

I must also reiterate that swallowing tablets of the enzymes SOD, catalase and glutathione peroxidase cannot confer beneficial antioxidant activity because the preparations are broken down and inactivated in the stomach. In my view manufacturers should be more scientific in their approach and produce natural products whose effects are scientifically credible. Surely we should strive to make effective products from natural ingredients and support these with sound pharmacological and clinical data?

Developing more natural products

Through these pages I'd like to pass on my own experiences to manufacturers of natural products. I would like to encourage them to establish which are the active components of their products and promote these in a scientific manner. I can strongly recommend the use of the methods employed in the manufacture of Bio Harmony for the extraction of active principles and I should be happy for other manufacturers to follow my lead. So many people want natural products instead of synthetic drugs (that may be ineffective or even damaging) so let's produce items that we can be sure will have the best possible effect.

Although Bio Harmony is an entirely natural product, the method I have established for its production may be technically described as a drug delivery system (DDS).[85-87] This does not, of course, mean that Bio Harmony should be considered as any sort of medicine. Far from it: Bio Harmony is a special food form, full of entirely natural food ingredients. I choose to use to the words 'drug delivery system' to highlight the very special care taken in the production of the material.

I should like to encourage others to develop DDSs in recognition of their potential to extract the very best nutritional value from natural ingredients. It is encouraging to me that similar findings on bioavailability are now being discussed at medical, chemical and agricultural science symposia. Other researchers are collecting evidence that bioactive low molecular weight compounds and peptides are produced from food protein in the presence of protease enzymes or as a by-product of brewing certain protein-containing foods such as soya beans.[88] These active components may be described in scientific terms as macrophage-activating peptide, angiotensin-transforming, enzyme-inhibitory peptide, cyclo peptide (His-Pro) and others.[88-90] It has also been reported that heat treatment increases the production of some of these bioactive substances,[88] as we found ourselves during the production of Bio Harmony.

I find it most encouraging that other scientists should publish papers in broad support of the method I devised to release the pharmacological potential of natural products. Personally I obtained my inspiration from the traditional methods of both China and Japan. Since ancient times herbs heated in pottery vessels and rice cooked in clay vessels have been used in the treatment of gastrointestinal complaints. In the modern jargon of today, this ancient tradition might feasibly be described as an empirically-derived oriental drug delivery system.

I have recently been investigating another natural product, a herbal mixture used in China for centuries. I have demonstrated that this mixture is strikingly effective in prolonging the lives of patients with malignancies, and am in the process of recording my findings. The mixture consists of five Chinese herbs: Bezoar Bovis, Kadinum, Rhei rhizoma, Hoelen and Arecae semen. Each of these is commonly sold in China and Japan for a variety of diseases, including cancers. I have established that individually they are ineffective, but if prepared together in a manner similar to Bio Harmony they do demonstrate a very marked effect. This increased potency of the materials provides further evidence that the drug delivery system described in this book is of exceptional value. It may be considered to enhance the bio-availability of pharmacologically active natural materials.

I will go so far as to suggest that if the Bio Harmony method of extraction is applied to other selected natural materials then these too will become far more effective in treating patients with oxygen radical- and lipid peroxide-related diseases. I can visualize the method in use for the benefit of mankind, employing a variety of Chinese and French herbs and a whole range of natural products and health foods currently available commercially throughout the world. It looks as though at last we have the key to unlock the door to release a myriad of hitherto unavailable health-giving natural materials. How wonderful to look forward to a world with safe, effective natural treatments that can take the place of the frightening synthetic chemical drugs of today.

Bibliography

1. McCord, J.M. and Fridovich, I. Superoxide dismutase. An enzymatic function for erythrocuprein (hemocuprein), J. Biol. Chem. 244:6049-55, (1969).

2. McCord, J.M., Keele, B.B. and Fridovich, I. An enzyme-based theory of obligate anaerobiosis: The physiological function of superoxide dismutase. Proc. Natl. Acad. Sci. USA 68:1024-27, (1971).

3. Yagi, K. A Simple fluorometric assay for lipoperoxide in blood plasma. Biochem. Med. 15:212-16, (1976).

4. Sato, Y., Hotta, N., Sakamoto, N., Matsuoka, S., Ohishi, N. and Yagi, K. Lipid peroxide level in plasma of diabetic patients. Biochem. Med. 21:104-7, (1979).

5. Nishigaki, I., Hagihara, M., Hiramatsu, M., Izawa, I. and Yagi, K. Effect thermal injury on lipid peroxide levels of rat. Biochem. Med. 24:185-89, (1980).

6. Yagi, K. Toxicity of lipid peroxides in processed foods. In: Biochemical Reviews, Golden Jubilee Volume L. H.R. Cama, N. Appaji Rao and R.N. Sharma, eds. The Society of Biological Chemists, India, 42-46, (1980).

7. Yagi, K., Matsuoka, S., Ohkawa, H., Ohishi, N., Takeuchi, Y.K. and Sakai, H. Lipoperoxide level of the retina of chick embryo exposed to high concentration of oxygen. Clin. Chim. Acta 80:355-60, (1977).

8. Yagi, Y., Matsuda, M. and Yagi, K. Formation of lipoperoxide in isolated sciatic nerve by chinoform-ferric chelate. Separatum Experienta 32:905-6, (1976).

9. Boxer, LA., Oliver, J.M., Spielberg, S.P., Allen, J.M.,

Schulman, B.A. and Schulman, J.D. Protection of granulocytes by vitamin E in glutathione synthetase deficiency. N. Engl. J. Med. 301:901-5, (1979).

10. Niwa, Y. and Tsutsui, D. Studies on carcinogenicity in heavy smokers – with special reference to the ratio of generation of oxygen intermediates to superoxide dismutase activity. Saishinigaku (in Jap.) 38:1450-58 (1983).

11. Niwa, Y., Miyake, S., Sakane, T., Shingu, M. and Yokoyama, M. Auto-oxidative damage in Behcet's disease — endothelial cell damage following the elevated oxygen radicals generated by stimulated neutrophils. Clin. Exp. Immunol. 49:247-55, (1982).

12. Niwa, Y. and Sohmiya, K. Enhanced neutrophilic functions in mucocutaneous lymph node syndrome, with special reference to the possible role of increased oxygen intermediate generation in the pathogenesis of coronary thromboarteritis. J. Pediatr. 104:56-60, (1984).

13. Niwa, Y., Sakane, T., Shingu, M. and Yokoyama, M.M. Effect of stimulated neutrophils from the synovial fluid of patients with rheumatoid arthritis on lymphocytes — a possible role of increased oxygen radicals generated by the neutrophils. J. Clin. Immunol. 3:228-40, (1983).

14. Niwa, Y., Sakane, T., Shingu, M., Yanagida, I., Komura, J. and Miyachi, Y. Neutrophil-generated active oxygens in linear IgA bullous dermatosis. Arch. Dermatol. 121:73-8, (1985).

15. Niwa, Y., Sakane, T., Shingu, M. and Miyachi, Y. Role of stimulated neutrophils from patients with systemic lupus erythematosus in tissue injury, with special reference to serum factors and increased active oxygen species generated by neutrophils. Inflammation 9:163-72, (1985).

16. Miyachi, Y., Uchida, K., Komura, U., Asada, Y. and Niwa, Y. Auto-oxidative damages in cement dermatitis. Arch. Dermatol. Res. 277:288-92, (1985).

17. Niwa, Y., Sakane, T. and Miyachi, Y. Dissociation of the inhibitory effect of dapsone on the generation of oxygen intermediates — in comparison with that of colchicine and various scavengers. Biochem. Pharmacol. 33:2355-60, (1984).

18. Niwa, Y., Sakane, T., Miyachi, Y., Kanoh, T. and Somiya, K. Decrease in generation of reactive oxygen species by neutrophils from patients with infectious mononucleosis: role of suppressor T lymphocytes. *Blood* 64:994-99, (1984).

19. Niwa, Y., Sakane, T., Miyachi, Y. and Ozaki, M. Oxygen metabolism in phagocytes of leprotic patients: enhanced endogenous superoxide dismutase activity and hydroxyl radical generation by clofazimine. *J. Clin. Microbiol.* 20:837-42, (1984).

20. Niwa, Y., Sakane, T., Somiya, K. and Miyachi, Y. Decreased oxygen radical generation by neutrophils from patients with measles presumably owing to activation of suppressor T lymphocytes. *J. Clin. Microbiol.* 21:318-22, (1985).

21. Niwa, Y., Kanoh, T., Sakane, T., Soh, H., Kawai, S. and Miyachi, Y. Detection of enhanced lipid peroxide levels in patients with inflammatory skin diseases. *J. Clin. Biochem. Nutr.* 2:245-51, (1987).

22. Niwa, Y., Kanoh, T., Sakane, T., Soh, H., Kawai, S. and Miyachi, Y. The ratio of lipid peroxides to superoxide dismutase activity in the skin lesions of patients with severe skin diseases: an accurate prognostic indicator. *Life Sci.* 40:921-27, (1987).

23. Niwa, Y., Kasama, T., Kawai, S., Komura, J., Sakane, T., Kanoh, T. and Miyachi, Y. The effect of aging on cutaneous lipid peroxide levels and superoxide dismutase activity in guinea pigs and patients with burns. *Life Sci.* 42:351-56, (1988).

24. Niwa, Y., Somiya, K., Michelson, A.M. and Puget, K. Effect of liposomal-encapsulated superoxide dismutase on active oxygen-related human disorders. *Free Rad. Res. Comms.* 1:137-53, (1985).

25. Niwa, Y. and Miyachi, Y. Antioxidant action of natural health products and Chinese herbs. *Inflammation* 10:79-91, (1986).

26. Niwa, Y., Kanoh, T., Kasama, T. and Negishi, M. Activation of antioxidant activity in natural medicinal products by heating, brewing and lipophilization. A new drug delivery system. *Drugs Exptl. Clin. Res.*, 14:361-72 (1988).

27. Granger, D.N., Rutili, G. and McCord, J.M. Superoxide

radicals in feline intestinal ischemia. *Gastroenterology* 81:22-29, (1981).

28. McCord, J.M. and Roy, R.S. The pathophysiology of superoxide: roles in inflammation and ischemia. *Can. J. Physiol. Pharmacol.* 60:1346-52, (1982).

29. Burton, K.P., McCord, J.M. and Ghai, G. Myocardial alterations due to free-radical generation. *Am. J. Physiol.* 247:H776-H783, (1984).

30. Zigler, J.S. Jr., Bodaness, R.S., Gery, I. and Kinoshita, J.H. Effects of lipid peroxidation products on the rat lens in organ culture: a possible mechanism of cataract initiation in retinal degenerative disease. *Arch. Biochem. Biophys.* 225: 149-56, (1983).

31. Hiramatsu, T., Hasegawa, Y., Hirata, K., Nishigaki, I. and Yagi K. Formation of lipoperoxide in the retina of rabbit exposed to high concentration of oxygen. *Separatum Experientia* 32:622-23, (1976).

32. Medeiros, M.H.G., Marchiori, P.E. and Bechara, E.J.H. Superoxide dismutase, glutathione peroxidase, and catalase activities in the erythrocytes of patients with intermittent acute porphyria. *Clin. Chem.* 28:242-43, (1982).

33. Farrington, J.A., Ebert, M., Land, E.J. and Fletcher, K. Bipyridylium quaternary salts and related compounds. V. Pulse radiolysis studies of the reaction of Paraquat radical with oxygen. Implications for the mode of action of bipyridyl herbicides. *Biochem. Biophys.* Acta 314:372-81, (1973).

34. Pyatak, P.S., Abuchowski, A. and Davis, F.F. Preparation of a polyethylene glycol: Superoxide dismutase adduct, and an examination of its blood circulating life and anti-inflammatory activity. *Res. Commun. Chem. Pathol. Pharmacol.* 29:113-27, (1980).

35. Fisher, H.K., Humphries, M. and Balls, R. Paraquat poisoning. Recovery from renal and pulmonary damage. *Ann. Intern. Med.* 75:731-36, (1971).

36. Ishida, R. and Takahashi, T. Increased DNA chain breakage by combined action of bleomycin and superoxide radical.

Biochem. Biophys. Res. Commun. 66:1432-38, (1975).

37. Sugiura, Y. and Suzuki, T. Nucleotide sequence specificity of DNA cleavage by iron-bleomycin. *J. Biol. Chem.* 257:10544-46, (1982).

38. Ferrans, V.J. Anthracycline cardiotoxicity. *Adv. Exp. Med. Biol.* 161:519-32, (1983).

39. Von Hoff, D.D., Rozencweig, M., Layard, M., Slavik, M. and Muggia, F.M. Daunomycin-induced cardiotoxicity in children and adults. *Am. J. Med.* 62:200-08, (1977).

40. Lefrak, E.A., Pitha, J., Rosenheim, S. and Gottlieb, J.A. A clinicopathologic analysis of adriamycin cardiotoxicity. *Cancer* 32:302-14, (1973).

41. Malaisse, W.J., Malaisse-Lagae, F., Sener, A. and Pipeleers, D.G. Determinants of the selective toxicity of alloxan to the pancreatic B cell. *Proc. Natl. Acad. Sci. USA* 79:927-30, (1982).

42. Grankvist, K., Marklund, S. and Täljedal, I.-B. Superoxide dismutase is a prophylactic against alloxan diabetes. *Nature* 294:158-60, (1981).

43. Heikkila, R.E., Winston, B., Cohen, G. and Barden, H. Alloxan-induced diabetes — evidence for hydroxyl radical as a cytotoxic intermediate. *Biochem. Pharmacol.* 25:1085-92, (1976).

44. Saito, Y., Ohishi, N. and Yagi, K. Protective effect of riboflavin on suppression of growth caused by oxidized oil. *J. Nutr. Sci. Vitaminol.* 25:17-21, (1981).

45. Kaneda, T., Sakai, H. and Ishii, S. Nutritive value or toxicity of highly unsaturated fatty acids (I and II). *J. Biochem.* 41:327-34, 1954; 42:561-68, (1955).

46. Tovar, L.R. and Kaneda, T. Comparative toxicity of secondary oxidation products in autoxidized methyl linoleate. *Yukagaku* 26:169-78, (1977).

47. Welsch, C.W. Enhancement of mammary tumorigenesis by dietary fat: Review of potential mechanisms. *Am. J. Clin. Nutr.* 45:192-202, (1987).

48. Michelson, A.M. Oxygen radicals. *Agents Actions (Suppl.)* 11:179-201, (1982).

49. Emerit, I. and Michelson, A.M. Mechanism of photosensi-

tivity in systemic lupus erythematosus patients. *Proc. Natl. Acad. Sci.* USA 78:2537-40, (1981).

50. Emerit, I. and Michelson, A.M. Chromosome instability in human and murine autoimmune disease: anticlastogenic effect of superoxide dismutase. *Acta Physiol. Scand.* 429:59-65, (1980).

51. Emerit, I., Housset, E. and Feingold, J. Chromosomal breakage and scleroderma: studies in family members. *J. Lab. Clin. Med.* 88: 81-86, (1976).

52. Scot, D. The effect of irradiated plasma on normal human chromosomes and its relevance to the long-lived lymphocyte hypothesis. *Cell Tissue Kinet.* 2:295-305, (1969).

53. Nordenson, I. Chromosome breaks in Werner's syndrome and their prevention in vitro by radical-scavenging enzymes. *Hereditas* 87:151-54, (1977).

54. Emerit, I., Loeper, J. and Chomette, G. Superoxide dismutase in the treatment of post-radiotherapeutic necrosis and of Crohn's disease. *Bull. Europ. Physiopath. Resp.* 17 (Suppl.):287-88, (1981).

55. Nishigaki, I., Hagihara, M., Maseki, M., Tomoda, Y., Nagayama, K., Nakashima, T. and Yagi, K. Effect of linoleic acid hydroperoxide on uptake of low density lipoprotein by cultured smooth muscle cells from rabbit aorta. *Biochem. Intern.* 8:501-08, (1984).

56. Yagi, K. Increased serum lipid peroxides initiate atherogenesis. *Bio Essays* 1:58-60, (1984).

57. Nighigaki, I., Hagihara, M., Tsunekawa, H., Maseki, M. and Yagi, K. Lipid peroxide levels of serum lipoprotein fractions of diabetic patients. *Biochem. Med.* 25:373-78, (1981).

58. Suematsu, T., Kamada, T., Abe, H., Kikuchi, S. and Yagi, K. Serum lipoperoxide level in patients suffering from liver diseases. *Clin. Chim. Acta* 79:267-70, (1977).

59. Maseki, M., Nishigaki, I., Hagihara, M., Tomoda, Y. and Yagi, K. Lipid peroxide levels and lipid content of serum lipoprotein fractions of pregnant subjects with or without pre-eclampsia. *Clin. Chim. Acta* 115:155-61, (1981).

60. Gregory, E.M. and Fridovich, I. Induction of superoxide

dismutase by molecular oxygen, J. *Bacteriol*. 114:543-48, (1973).

61. Tanaka, K. and Sugahara, K. Role of superoxide dismutase in defense against SO_2 toxicity and an increase in superoxide dismutase activity with SO_2 fumigation, *Plant Cell Physiol*. 21:601-11, (1980).

62. Rabinowitch, H.D., Clare, D.A., Crapo, J.D. and Fridovich, I. Positive correlation between superoxide dismutase and resistance to Paraquat toxicity in the green alga chlorella sorokiniana. *Arch. Biochem. Biophys*. 225:640-648, (1983).

63. Sugiura, K., Abe, M., Inasaka, H., Ueda, H., Harano, K. and Adachi, T. Studies on superoxide dismutase in human skin (4). Contents of superoxide dismutase and lipid peroxide in keloid, hypertrophic scar and scar. *Jap. J. Dermatol*. (in Jap.) 96:171-74, (1986).

64. Michelson, A.M., Puget, K., Durosay, P. and Bonneau, J.C. Clinical aspects of the dosage of erythrocuprein. In: Superoxide and Superoxide Dismutases. A.M. Michelson, J.M. McCord and I. Fridovich, eds. *Academic Press*, 467-99, (London, 1977).

65. Niwa, Y., Kasama, Miyachi, Y. and Kanoh, T. Neutrophil chemotaxis, phagocytonis and parameters of reactive oxygen species in human ageing: cross-sectional and longitudinal studies. *Am. J. Pathol*., [in press], (1989).

66. Heinecke, J.W., Baker, L., Rosen, H. and Chait, A. Superoxide-mediated modification of low density lipoprotein by arterial smooth muscle cells. *J. Clin. Invest*. 77:757-61, (1986).

67. Hiramatsu, K., Rosen, H., Heinecke, J.W., Wolfbauer, G. and Chait, A. Superoxide initiates oxidation of low density lipoprotein by human monocytes. *Arteriosclerosis* 7:55-60, (1987).

68. Goldstein, J.L., Basu, S.K. and Brown, M.S. Receptor-mediated endocytosis of low-density lipoprotein in cultured cells. *Methods Enzymol*. 98:241-60, (1983).

69. Niwa, Y. Superoxide dismutase. *Biomedicine & Therapeutics* (in Jap.) 19:730-34, (1987).

70. Baillet, F., Housset, M., Michelson, A.M. and Puget, K.

Treatment of radiofibrosis with liposomal superoxide dismutase. Preliminary results of 50 cases. *Free Rad. Res. Comms.* 1:387-94, (1986).

71. Michelson, A.M. and Puget, K. Cell penetration by exogenous superoxide dismutase. *Acta Physiol. Scand.* (Suppl.) 492:67-80, (1980).

72. Dangeon, O. and Michelson, A.M. Cellular fixation, penetration and intracellular localization of glutathione peroxidase and liposomal forms of the enzyme. *Mol. Physiol.* 3:35-41, (1983).

73. Michelson, A.M., Puget, K., Perdereau, B. and Barbaroux, C. Scintigraph studies on the localization of liposomal superoxide dismutase injected into rabbits. *Mol. Physiol.* 1:71-84, (1981).

74. Somiya, K., Niwa, Y., Shimoda, K., Fukami, S., Puget, K and Michelson, A.M. Treatment with liposomal superoxide dismutase of patients with Kawasaki disease. *In*: Superoxide and Superoxide Dismutase in *Chemistry, Biology and Medicine*. G. Rotilio, 513-16, ed. Elsevier Science Publishers, Amsterdam, (1986).

75. Michelson, A.M. Oxygen radicals in chemistry and biology. *In*: Proceedings Third International Conference. W. Bors, M. Saran and D. Tait, [eds.] 986-87, Walter de Gruyter, Berlin, New York, (1984).

76. Michelson, A.M. Medical aspects of liposomal-encapsulated superoxide dismutase. Life Chemistry Reports 6:1-142, (1987).

77. Niwa, Y. Investigation of skin tissue activating factors, enzyme activities and influence of bioactive substances on cell membrane. *Fragrance Journal* (in Jap.) 16:37-48, (1988).

78. Dall'Acqua, F. and Caffieri, S. Recent and selected aspects of furocoumarin photochemistry and photobiology. *Photo. Med. Photo. Biol.* 10:1-46, (1988).

79. Tomita, Y. and Seiji, M. Inactivation mechanism of tyrosinase in mouse melanoma. *J. Dermatol.* 4:245-49, (1977).

80. Negishi, M., Fukushima, T., Tabata, M., Sato, H., Kobayashi, K., Ide, H. and Takahashi, T. Clinical study on the effect of

antioxidant analogs in collagen disease (in Jap.) *Japanese Inflammation*, [in press], (1989).

81. Hill, T.J., Blyth, W.A. and Harbour, D.A. Trauma to the skin causes recurrence of herpes simplex in the mouse. *J. Gen. Virol.* 39:21-28, (1978).

82. Hill, T.J. Mechanisms involved in recurrent herpes simplex. In: *The Human Herpesviruses*. A.J. Nahmias, *et al.*, eds. Elsevier, Amsterdam, 241-244, (1981).

83. Blyth, W.A., Hill, T.J., Field, H.J. and Harbour, D.A. Reactivation of herpes simplex virus infection by ultraviolet light and possible involvement of prostaglandins. *J. Gen. Virol.* 33:547-50, (1976).

84. Sato, H., Takahashi, T., Ide, H., Fukushima, T., Tabata, M., Sekine, F., Kobayashi, K., Negishi, M. and Niwa, Y. Antioxidant activity of synovial fluid, hyaluronic acid, and 2 subcomponents of hyaluronic acid. Synovial fluid scavenging effect is enhanced in rheumatoid arthritis patients. *Arthritis Rheum.*, 31:63-71, (1988).

85. Roseman, T.J. and Mandorf, S.Z., eds. *Controlled Release Delivery Systems*. Marcel Dekker, Inc., New York and Basel, (1983).

86. Chien, Y.W. Novel drug delivery systems: fundamentals, developmental concepts, biomedical assessments. *Drugs and the Pharmaceutical Sciences*, Vol. 14, Marcel Dekker, Inc., New York and Basel, (1982).

87. Smalen, V.F. and Ball, L.A., eds. Drug Product Design and Performance. *Controlled Drug Bioavailability*, Vol. 1. John Wiley & Sons, New York, (1984).

88. Ninomiya, M., Kawai, M. and Yanagisawa, T. Detection of the presence of bioactive peptide cyclo (His-Pro) in foods (in Jap.). In: *Abstract paper for the Annual Meeting of the Agricultural Chemical Society of Japan*, 267, Kyoto, 1987.

89. Chiba, H. and Yoshikawa, M. Biologically functional peptides from food proteins: New opioid peptides from milk proteins. In: *Protein Tailoring for Food and Medical Uses*. R.G. Feeney and J.R. Whitaker, eds. Marcel Dekker, Inc., New York and Basel, 123-53, (1986).

90. Yanagisawa, T., Ninomiya, M. and Ikeda, T. Production of bioactive peptide cyclo (His-Pro) from brewed foods during their storage (in Jap.). In: *Abstract paper for the Annual Meeting of the Agricultural Chemical Society of Japan*, 563, Kyoto, (1986).

91. Rosen, H. and Klebanoff, S.J. Role of iron and ethylenediaminetetraaceitc acid in the bactericidal activity of a superoxide anion-generating system. *Biochem. Biophys. Acta* 208:512-29, (1981).

92. Ambruso, D.R. and Johnston, R.B. Jr. Lactoferrin enhanced hydroxyl radical production by human neutrophils, neutrophil particulate fractions, and an enzymatic generating system. *J. Clin. Invest.* 67:352-60, (1981).

Appendix

	tissue	lipid peroxide levels (nmol/mg protein)	SOD activity (unit/mg protein)
blood cells	erythrocytes	0.08±0.02 (62.3±11 nmol/g Hb)	89±6.6
	T lymphocytes	1.26±0.08	5.8±0.7
	B lymphocytes	0.91±0.07	3.1±0.5
	monocytes	0.48±0.03	1.5±0.1
	macrophages	0.44±0.03	1.2±0.2
	neutrophils	0.59±0.04	2.0±0.4
	platelets	0.96±0.07	3.9±0.6
skin, muscle	epidermis/dermis	0.72±0.07	8.4±1.2
	dermis/fat tissue	0.61±0.06	6.5±1.8
	muscle	0.55±0.05	2.9±0.5
internal organs	liver	1.12±0.10	66.7±9.6
	kidney	1.04±0.10	60.2±8.9
	spleen	0.84±0.07	41.2±5.3
	lung	0.79±0.07	37.5±4.5
	pancreas	0.66±0.05	24.6±3.1
	stomach	0.56±0.05	9.6±1.1
	small intestine	0.53±0.04	9.3±1.2
	colon	0.40±0.03	6.1±0.8

Table A1 Lipid peroxide levels and SOD activity in healthy blood cells, tissues and organs

	markedly effective	effective	slightly effective	no effect	undecided	% efficacy
Behcet's disease (18)	0	4	2	8	4	43%
RA (rheumatoid arthritis) 1) evaluated by Lansbury index (77)	3	10	4	55	5	24%
2) evaluated mainly by morning stiffness (77)	6	33	12	20	6	72%
3) the combination therapy with sulbenicillin (or cefaclor) (60)	8	25	9	12	6	78%
Crohn's disease (6)	0	3	1	2	0	67%
progressive systemic sclerosis (PSS) and polymyositis (10)	1	3	1	4	1	56%
Raynaud's disease (14)	2	4	2	5	1	62%
hepatitis (13)	3	4	0	5	1	58%
diabetes (7)	0	2	1	4	0	43%
nephritis (11)	4	2	0	5	0	55%
undefined general complaints (general malaise, cold fingers and toes, lumbago, shoulder stiffness, constipation) (44)	0	14	13	12	5	69%
reduced sexual capacity (11)	0	4	2	3	2	67%
hangover (13)	0	5	2	3	3	70%
irregular periods (12)	0	5	3	3	1	73%
arteria coronaria insufficiency (25)	2	4	4	10	5	50%
cerebral arterial sclerosis (30)	2	5	4	13	6	46%
cerebrovascular thrombosis (7)	0	0	1	1	5	50%
myocardial infarction (8)	0	1	1	1	5	67%
prevention of repeat attacks of cerebrovascular thrombosis (15)	0	13	1	1	0	93%
prevention of recurrence of myocardial infarction (13)	0	10	1	1	1	92%
atopic dermatitis with severe lesions in exposed area (13)	0	2	2	6	3	40%
chilblains (16)	1	6	1	6	2	59%
sun-burn dermatitis (9)	0	2	1	4	2	43%
common wart (12)	3	4	2	3	0	75%
burn (III - IV grade) or wound with ulcer lesions (15)	3	5	1	5	1	64%
preventing keloid scar formation in susceptible people (7)	0	2	2	2	1	67%
freckles (79)	16	22	14	21	6	71%

Parentheses ( ) denote the number of cases tested.

Table A2 Clinical effect of Bio Harmony in various disorders

Index